This textbook gives a broad, but conci⁣s̶⁣e̶ ⁣ ⁣ ⁣ ⁣ ⁣ ⁣ ⁣ ⁣ ⁣ ⁣ ⁣ ⁣ ⁣ ⁣ ⁣ ⁣ ⁣ ⁣ ⁣g and manipulation, suitable for undergradua⁣t⁣e⁣ ⁣,⁣ graduate students, or others learning gene cloning for the first time. Assuming only general elementary biochemical knowledge, it stresses the concepts underlying particular types of cloning vectors and illustrates these concepts by using specific examples, rather than simply presenting a mass of detailed lists and vector maps.

The book starts by describing the principles behind cloning DNA in *E. coli*, the enzymes used, the range of cloning vectors available, and methods for screening libraries to find particular clones. The author shows how PCR can be used as an alternative, or complementary, approach. He then goes on to describe how sequences – once they have been cloned and identified – can be exploited by site-directed mutagenesis and overexpression. The book finishes with a detailed presentation of the genetic manipulation of other organisms, including other bacteria, yeast and other fungi, *Chlamydomonas,* plants, insects, and mammals.

This concise, readable account will be invaluable for all those wanting to understand the concepts and principles behind these fundamental biological techniques.

GENE CLONING
AND
MANIPULATION

GENE CLONING AND MANIPULATION

CHRISTOPHER HOWE

Department of Biochemistry
University of Cambridge

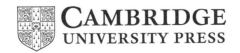
CAMBRIDGE
UNIVERSITY PRESS

Published by the Press Syndicate of the University of Cambridge
The Pitt Building, Trumpington Street, Cambridge CB2 1RP
40 West 20th Street, New York, NY 10011-4211, USA
10 Stamford Road, Oakleigh, Melbourne 3166, Australia

First published 1995

Printed in the United States of America

Library of Congress Cataloging-in-Publication Data
Howe, Christopher, 1959–
Gene cloning and manipulation / Christopher Howe.
p.   cm.
Includes bibliographical reference and index.
ISBN 0-521-40341-3 (hbk.).– ISBN 0-521-40700-1 (pbk.)
1. Molecular cloning.   I. Title.
QH442.2.H69   1995
575.1'0724 – dc20   94-42638
                                                                          CIP

A catalog record for this book is available from the British Library.

ISBN 0-521-40341-3 Hardback
ISBN 0-521-40700-1 Paperback

Contents

CHAPTER **3**
Other Vector Systems for *E. Coli*   43

CHAPTER **4**
Making Libraries   67

Preface

This book grew out of sets of lectures given to undergraduates taking courses in Biochemistry and Molecular Biology, and Medical Sciences. I hope it will be useful to people studying a range of biological subjects. I have tried to concentrate throughout on the general principles underlying the subject rather than to give overwhelmingly detailed accounts of vector systems and practical instructions. For those, there are more detailed books, reviews, catalogues, and lab manuals. I am grateful to the many friends and colleagues who have helped in the production of this book by reading sections (and in some cases the whole thing!) or in other ways. In particular, I should like to thank Janet Allen, Alison Baker, Adrian Barbrook, Alison Franklin, Hilary and Tony Larkum, and Saul Purton. I am also grateful to Robin Smith of Cambridge University Press for his advice and encouragement throughout the exercise, and to Robert Sugar and Dorothy Duncan of Bookworks for their help in the book's production.

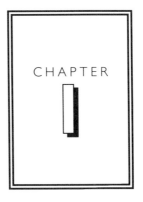

CHAPTER

1

The Tools
for the Job

1.1 INTRODUCTION

Cloning and manipulating genes requires the ability to cut, modify, and join genetic material (usually DNA but sometimes RNA), and to check the parameters, such as size, of the molecules that are being manipulated. We will assume a knowledge of the structure of the materials involved – DNA, RNA, and so on – and start by describing the tools available for manipulating them. Almost all the tools involved are enzymes that have important physiological roles in cells. To understand why they are useful for our purposes, we should be aware of their normal roles, too.

The choice of which enzyme is used for a particular purpose depends mainly on two considerations:

1. How easy (i.e., inexpensive) is it to purify? This will be determined by its abundance in the cell and by how easy it is to separate it from other undesirable activities.

2. How well does it do the job? This will depend upon its specificity ("accuracy") and specific activity ("speed"), as well as the details of the reaction which it catalyses.

Other factors, such as stability, are also important.

1

Techniques of genetic manipulation can be applied to the production of the enzymes for genetic engineering. It is possible to use cloned genes to prepare large quantities of these enzymes more easily, as well as to modify the genes to "improve" their function, perhaps by altering slightly the properties of the enzymes they encode.

1. 2 CUTTING

Enzymes that break down nucleic acids are called nucleases. Those that break down RNA are called ribonucleases, or RNases, and those that break down DNA are called deoxyribonucleases, or DNases. There are two ways of breaking down a linear nucleic acid molecule: dismantling it bit by bit from the ends, or breaking it into pieces by cutting within the molecule. The former is called exonucleolytic activity (Greek *exo* = outside) and the latter endonucleolytic activity (Greek *endon* = within). Don't fall into the trap of thinking that *endo*nucleases work from the *ends* in! For cutting nucleic acid molecules into pieces, we will therefore need endonucleases, and the most widely used ones are the restriction endonucleases.

1. 2. 1 Restriction endonucleases

Restriction endonucleases are part of the natural defence mechanisms of bacteria against incoming DNA, which may be from viruses or plasmids from a foreign population of cells. These enzymes were first recognized by their ability to *restrict* the growth of certain viruses in certain strains of *E. coli* and were named accordingly. (The verb *restrict* is now widely used by molecular biologists to mean "cut with a restriction endonuclease".) They are associated with modifying enzymes, which methylate the DNA. Methylation protects the DNA from cleavage by endonucleases, and this stops the cell from degrading its own DNA. Invading DNA that has not been correctly methylated will be degraded, unless it can be modified by the cell's methylating enzymes quickly enough – which happens rarely.

DNA, once modified, remains protected even after replication. This is because semiconservative replication of a molecule methylated on both strands results in two daughter molecules that are hemimethylated (i.e., methylated on one strand), and hemimethylation is sufficient to confer endonuclease protection. The other strand will be then be modified before replication takes place again.

Three types of restriction-modification systems are recognized. These are called classes (or types) I, II, and III, and their key properties are summarized in Table 1.1. All the enzymes recognize particular DNA sequences, but only the Class II endonucleases cut within those recognition sequences. The recognition sites for a number of Class II enzymes are given in Table 1.2. These enzymes often make a "staggered" cut to leave molecules that, although primarily double-stranded, have short single-stranded ends. These are called *sticky* ends. Depending on the enzyme, either the 5' end or the 3' end may be left single-stranded. The molecules generated have a phosphate group on the 5' end and a hydroxyl group on the 3' end. A small number of Class II enzymes cut just outside their recognition sites; for example, *Mbo*II cuts 7 nucleotides 3' to its recognition site of -GAAGA-. Some cleave within their recognition sites, but at degenerate sequences; for example, *Mam*I cuts at -GATNN'NNATC-. Nevertheless,

TABLE I.I Characteristics of restriction and modification systems

	CLASS I	CLASS II	CLASS III
Composition	Multienzyme complex with R (endonuclease), M (methylase), and S (specificity) subunits, e.g., as R_2M_2S	Separate enzymes; endonuclease is a homodimer, methylase a monomer	M subunit provides specificity; on its own, functions as methylase; as heterodimer with R subunit, functions as methylase-endonuclease
Cofactors	Mg^{2+}, ATP, SAM (needed for cleavage as well as methylation)	Mg^{2+}, SAM (for methylation only)	Mg^{2+}, ATP (for cleavage), SAM (needed for methylation; stimulates cleavage)
Recognition sites	Asymmetric, bipartite, may be degenerate. E.g., EcoK (AACN$_6$GTGC)	Symmetric, may be bipartite, may be degenerate (Table 1.2)	Asymmetric, uninterrupted, 5–6 nt long. E.g., EcoP15 - CAGCAG. 2 copies in opposite orientation but not necessarily adjacent needed for cleavage; 1 for methylation
Cleavage	Variable distance (100–1,000 nt) from recognition site	Within recognition site, except for Class IIs (shifted cleavage), which cleaves outside, at a defined distance	25–27 nt from recognition site
Number of systems	Several, grouped into a few families. E.g., K, includes EcoB, EcoD, EcoK, and others	Hundreds	Few

SAM = S-adenosyl methionine

these enzymes are still recognizably Class II on the basis of their biochemical properties. Except in the special cases just noted, all DNA molecules resulting from cutting with a given Class II enzyme will have the same sequence at their ends. That will not be true with the Class I and III enzymes, as they cut outside their recognition sites. Because molecules cut with a given Class II enzyme generally have the same ends, such molecules can base-pair with each other and, as we shall see, can be covalently joined by a DNA ligase. Some Class II enzymes give clean cuts rather than staggered ones, cutting both strands at the same place (see Table 1.2). This gives double-stranded or *blunt* ends on the molecules. That is not a problem, since blunt-ended molecules can also be joined by ligase. The following features of cleavage by Class II enzymes are also important:

1. **Recognition sites generally read the same on both strands** (as long as the same polarity, e.g., 5' to 3') is read. Such sequences are often described as *palin-*

TABLE 1.2 **Examples of recognition sequences of Class II restriction endonucleases**

*Apa*I	G GGCC'C C'CCGG G	*Aha*III	TTT'AAA AAA'TTT
*Bam*HI	G'GATC C C CTAG'G	*Bgl*II	A'GATC T T CTAG'A
*Bsp*120I	G'GGCC C C CCGG'C	*Dpn*I	GA'TC CT'AG
*Dra*I	TTT'AAA AAA'TTT	*Eco*RI	G'AATT C C TTAA'G
*Hinc*II	GTPy'PuAC CAPu'PyTG	*Hind*III	A'AGCT T T TCGA'A
*Hpa*II	C'CG G G GC'C	*Mae*III	'GTNAC CANTG'
*Not*I	GC'GGCC GC CG CCGG'CG	*Pvu*II	CAG'CTG GTC'GAC
*Sal*I	G'TCGA C C AGCT'G	*Sau*3A	'GATC CTAG'
*Sph*I	G CATG'C C'GTAC G	*Taq*I	T'CG A A GC'T
*Xba*I	T'CTAG A A GATC'T		

' = cleavage site; N = any nucleotide; Py and Pu = pyrimidine and purine nucleotides respectively.

dromes. It is not necessary for recognition sequences to be palindromic for all molecules cut with the same enzyme to be able to reanneal, although it does increase the number of configurations in which reassociation can take place. For example, Figure 1.1 shows how two molecules cut with the enzyme *Hind*III (recognition sequence -A'AGCTT-) can reanneal, with either end of the right-hand molecule able to anneal with either end of the left-hand one. Two molecules cut with an enzyme with a nonpalindromic recognition sequence could also reanneal, but only one end of the right-hand molecule would be capable of annealing to the left-hand molecule.

2. Most enzymes have recognition sites of 4 or 6 bases. If all bases occurred with equal frequencies (both in the DNA to be cut and in the enzyme recognition sites) and at random, a particular 4-nucleotide motif would be expected to occur on average once every 4^4 (i.e., 256) nucleotides. So the average length of fragments generated by enzymes with such sites would be 256 bases. Similarly, enzymes with a 6-base-pair recognition sequence would generate fragments

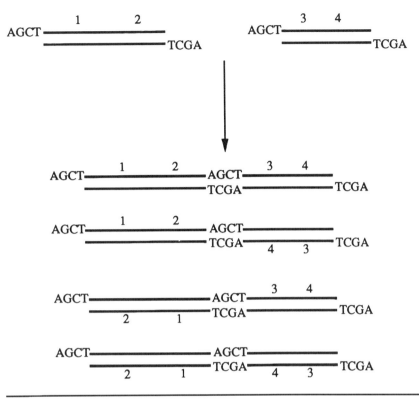

Figure 1.1 **Annealing of two molecules cut with *Hind*III.** I, 2, 3, and 4 represent arbitrary points on the molecules. Note that the right-hand molecule can anneal in two possible orientations to either end of the left-hand one because of the palindromic nature of the *Hind*III cleavage site.

with an average size of 4^6 (i.e., 4096) bases. In practice, that does not happen, for the following reasons:

a. The bases do not occur with equal frequencies in the recognition sites.

b. The bases do not occur with equal frequencies in the DNA to be cut, and the frequencies can vary over the genome.

c. The bases do not occur at random; for example, certain dinucleotides are favoured and others avoided. The degree of nonrandomness often varies over a genome.

3. Different enzymes can recognize the same sequence. For example, *Dra*I and *Aha*III both recognize and cut at -TTT'AAA-. They are said to be *isoschizomers.* Enzymes with the same recognition sequence don't necessarily cut at the same position within it, though. For example, *Apa*I recognizes and cuts at -GGGCC'C-, whereas *Bsp*120I recognizes and cuts at -G'GGCCC-.

4. Different enzymes can generate the same ends. For example, the enzyme *Sau*3AI produces the ends -GATC, and *Bam*HI does the same. That means that molecules produced by digestion with *Sau*3AI will be able to anneal and be ligated to molecules produced with *Bam*HI. Given that blunt-ended molecules can also be ligated, molecules cut with any enzymes that give blunt ends can be ligated. Notice, though, that ligation of molecules cut with different enzymes may not regenerate the original recognition sites used. It may also be possible to ligate – though at a lower efficiency – molecules whose sticky ends are nearly, but not fully, complementary.

5. Cutting can be influenced by other factors. The most important are

   a. methylation,

   b. the buffer used, and

   c. secondary structure in the substrate.

Methylation of bases in DNA may result from the modification activity of a restriction-modification system or from the activity of one of many independent methylases. Methylated bases commonly encountered include N^6-methyladenine, 5-methylcytosine, 5-hydroxymethylcytosine, and N^4-methylcytosine. Restriction enzymes will generally not cut molecules where specific bases within their recognition sites are methylated. This is the basis of a cell's protection of its own DNA. Methylation at other positions within the recognition site may not affect cleavage, and for some enzymes, methylation at other positions may actually be required for cleavage. For example, cleavage by *Bam*HI is inhibited by methylation at the internal C of the -GGATCC- recognition site but not by methylation of the other C or the A, whereas cleavage by *Apy*I is inhibited by methylation of the first C of its recognition site (-CCAGG- or -CCTGG-) but requires methylation of the second C.

The specificity of some enzymes is affected by the buffer used. For example, the enzyme *Eco*RI normally cuts at the sequence -GAATTC-, but in the presence of glycerol at concentrations greater than 5% v/v, the specificity is relaxed, and cutting can take place at -AATT- or -PuPuATPyPy-. That is often referred to as *star* activity, denoted *Eco*RI*. The extent of cutting can be modified by certain compounds. One example is ethidium bromide, shown in Figure 1.2. This molecule, which is also used for visualizing nucleic acids in gels (see Section 1.6.3), can be intercalated (inserted) between the bases in a double-stranded DNA molecule. That interferes with the action of restriction endonucleases, allowing cutting in one strand only.

Some sites are cut much less efficiently than others within the same molecule. This may be due to secondary structures in the DNA that interfere with recognition or cleavage by the endonuclease.

6. Enzyme activities are measured in *units*. A unit is the amount of an enzyme required to digest a standard amount (usually 1 microgram) of a standard type of DNA (often bacteriophage lambda, or a specified plasmid) in a given time (usually 1 hour) under given conditions (temperature, pH, etc.). Digesting DNA molecules containing many sites may therefore require more units of enzyme than the amount required to digest the same mass of a DNA containing fewer sites.

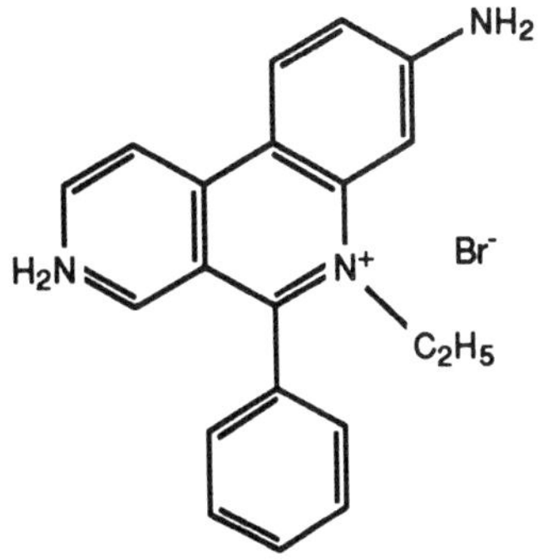

Figure 1.2 **Ethidium bromide.**

7. Restriction endonuclease preparations used for cloning must be free of other nucleases. If not, the ends of the molecules generated might be degraded by exonucleases, and reannealing would be prevented. Contaminating endonuclease activity would cut the molecules into fragments with no (or the wrong) single-stranded ends, which would cause a similar problem. Manufacturers therefore usually test enzyme preparations by incubating DNA with a large excess of the enzyme, then determining what fraction of the products can be religated and whether the religated molecules can still be cut with the enzyme. The higher the proportion of correct religation, the "cleaner" the enzyme preparation. Low levels of contaminating nucleases are not a problem in simple restriction enzyme mapping, though, and some suppliers sell *mapping* and *cloning* grades of the same enzyme.

8. Partial digestion may be useful. Sometimes we deliberately don't carry out digestion with a restriction enzyme to completion. For example, we might need to fragment total DNA (often called *genomic* DNA) prepared from an organism into pieces of roughly the same size, say 10 kb, so that every sequence in the organism is represented in the collection of 10-kb fragments. Simply cutting to completion with an enzyme with a 6-nucleotide recognition sequence and taking the fragments produced that are approximately 10 kb would not be suitable. A lot of the DNA would be cut into only smaller (or only larger) pieces and would never be represented in the 10-kb size class. A better method is to use an enzyme that cuts very frequently (e.g., at a 4-base-pair recognition site) but to adjust either the reaction time allowed or the ratio of enzyme to DNA in the reaction, so that only a few of the possible sites are cut. That way the average size of the fragments can be raised to 10 kb or whatever else is required, and if all sites have a more or less equal chance of being cut, all regions of the DNA can be represented among the 10-kb fragments (unless the distribution of sites in a particular region is grossly abnormal). This approach is very useful in constructing genomic libraries (see Section 4.2.1).

9. Cleavage sites can be determined using standard molecules. A selection of DNA molecules whose sequences are known completely are digested with the enzyme. Samples are also digested by combinations of the enzyme under test with others, which have known cleavage sites. The sizes of the fragments generated are measured by gel electrophoresis, and a computer analysis allows you to infer possible recognition sites from the sequences on the grounds that they are the only sites that would generate fragments of the observed sizes. More accurate measurement (to the exact number of nucleotides) of the sizes of molecules generated by digestion allows the actual cleavage site within the recognition sequence to be inferred. These accurate size measurements are also done electrophoretically, using the products of DNA sequencing reactions as size markers.

10. Nomenclature follows a simple convention. Once an enzyme has been characterized, it must be given a name. The convention is that names start with three letters (italicized): the first letter of the genus and the first two letters of the species of the source cells. Where relevant, they are followed by an indication of the strain and then a number (in Roman numerals) indicating which one of the enzymes from that strain the name refers to. For example, the enzymes *Eco*RI and *Eco*RII refer to the first and second activities isolated from strain R of *E. coli*. Often, names are abbreviated, so *Eco*RI is often referred to colloquially just as "RI" (pronounced "R-one"), *Bam*HI as "Bam", and so on.

I. 2. 2   DNase

In some instances, restriction endonucleases are unsuitable for cutting DNA. That might be so if the DNA has a very abnormal base composition, although such a wide variety of enzymes is now available, with so many recognition sites, that this is rarely a problem. A more common problem occurs when it is necessary to break DNA into a random collection of fragments as outlined in Section 1.2.1, but with a mean size of only a few hundred base pairs. (This is sometimes helpful in DNA sequencing projects; see Section 3.2.3). Partial digestion with a 4-nucleotide-recognizing enzyme is not suitable; nearly every site would have to be cut to get the required average size, and this would mean that some sequences would be represented only on fragments either much smaller or much larger than the size-range required. The problem can be avoided by using a DNase such as DNaseI, which has very little (and for this purpose essentially no) sequence specificity. Again, careful adjustment of either the enzyme-DNA ratio or the incubation time is necessary to ensure the optimal distribution of fragment sizes. One problem with the use of DNase is that the ends of the molecules produced do not have a unique single-stranded sequence. Also, not all the ends are blunt. This makes cloning of the fragments difficult, but the problem can be solved by rendering all the ends blunt with a suitable DNA polymerase, as described in Section 1.3.2.

I. 2. 3   Physical stress

In addition to enzymatic means, we can use physical shearing to cleave DNA at random. We can accomplish this in several ways; for example, we can simply stir a solution or force it through a narrow opening, such as a syringe needle or a pipette tip, or we can use sonication (which essentially provides high frequency vibrations). In practice, sonication is the preferred method, since it is the easiest to control and is often even more reproducible than DNaseI treatment. Different kinds of sonicator are available. In the simplest form, a metal probe is dipped into the solution and vibrates at high frequency. This has the disadvantage that the probe can be a source of cross-contamination between DNA preparations unless it is carefully cleaned. An alternative instrument is the cup-horn sonicator, in which the solution to be sonicated is retained in a tube that floats in a small volume of water. The probe is dipped into the surrounding water, and vibrations are transmitted through the water to the tube containing the sample. With shearing, as with DNase treatment, there is no control over the sequences at the ends of the fragments produced.

1.3 MODIFICATION

1.3.1 Phosphatases

Phosphatases are enzymes that hydrolytically remove phosphate groups from DNA molecules, replacing them with hydroxyl groups. The terminal phosphate groups left by restriction enzymes are needed for most ligation reactions, and the application of phosphatase in blocking unwanted ligation reactions will be described in Section 2.3.1. A widely used preparation comes from calf intestines, where the enzyme presumably has a digestive function. Shrimps are another source.

1.3.2 Polymerases

We will meet three classes of DNA or RNA polymerases: DNA-dependent DNA polymerases, RNA-dependent DNA polymerases, and DNA-dependent RNA polymerases.

1. DNA-dependent DNA polymerases. These enzymes synthesize a DNA strand in a 5'–3' direction using a DNA template. They can also have 5'–3' and 3'–5' exonuclease activities, and all these activities can be exploited in various ways. The preparations used come from bacteria, such as *E. coli* and *Thermus aquaticus*, and from bacteria infected with viruses such as T4 and T7. The *E. coli* enzyme that is widely used is DNA polymerase I, which normally has important roles in DNA repair and the replacement with DNA of the RNA primers used for DNA synthesis. The enzyme has 5'–3' polymerase, 3'–5' exonuclease (serving a proofreading function), and 5'–3' exonuclease activities. These are essentially located on different domains of the molecule. Cleavage with the protease subtilisin generates an N-terminal fragment of 35 kDa containing the 5'–3' exonuclease activity and a C-terminal one of 76 kDa with the polymerase and 3'–5' exonuclease activities (Figure 1.3). The 76-kDa piece is sometimes called the Klenow fragment, and the intact molecule the Kornberg enzyme.

The 5'–3' DNA polymerase activity allows a complementary DNA strand to be synthesized using a suitable template. This template might be a large piece of single-stranded DNA with a small primer annealed, or it might be a restriction fragment with a recessed 3' (i.e., overhanging 5') end. Incubation of either of these templates with DNA polymerase and the correct dideoxynucleoside triphosphates would result in the filling-in of the single-stranded region to produce a blunt-ended molecule. This is often called *end-filling*. Note that the 5'–3' exonucleolytic activity of the Kornberg enzyme could also produce such a molecule by degradation of the overhanging 5' end rather than by synthesis of its complement. A recessed 5' end cannot be rendered blunt by the polymerase activity, because synthesis would have to be in the 3'–5' direction, which is not

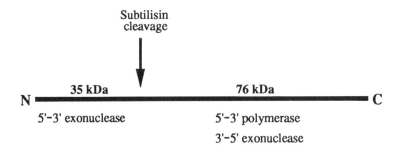

Figure 1.3 **DNA polymerase I.** The positions of the activities and the cleavage site of subtilisin are indicated.

possible. Again, the 3'–5' exonucleolytic activity could render the ends blunt by degradation. Rendering overhanging ends blunt by any of these means is termed *polishing* and is summarized in Figure 1.4.

The DNA polymerase from *Thermus aquaticus* (usually called *Taq* polymerase) is primarily used for synthesis of longer stretches of DNA, rather than for polishing ends. The source organism is an extreme thermophile, living in hot springs, and the enzyme is very resistant to heat denaturation. Indeed, its temperature optimum is $75°$–$80°C$. *Taq* polymerase is therefore particularly useful when reactions need to be carried out at high temperatures (such as when using a template that has a high G+C content with a lot of secondary structure that needs to be melted out by heating). This is often useful in DNA sequencing. Thermostable polymerases are also vitally important in the polymerase chain reaction (see Section 6.1.1), in which the reaction mixture containing the enzyme has to undergo repeated rounds of heating and cooling. Although the first widely used thermostable polymerase came from *T. aquaticus*, many are now available from other thermophilic bacteria.

The viral DNA polymerases are encoded in the viral genomes and are synthesized upon infection of *E. coli* cells. The polymerases are essential for replication of viral DNA in the absence of host DNA synthesis. T4 DNA polymerase has a particularly active 3'–5' exonuclease function (more than 200 times that of

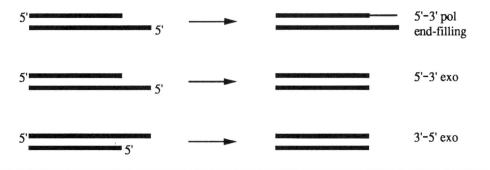

Figure 1.4 **Polishing overhanging ends using polymerase (pol) or exonuclease (exo) activity.** The thin line indicates DNA newly synthesized by polymerase activity.

the Klenow enzyme) and is especially useful in polishing up sticky ends. T7 DNA polymerase is widely used in DNA sequencing, where it generates fewer artifacts than does the Klenow fragment of DNA polymerase, probably as a result of higher processivity (i.e., a lower tendency to dissociate from the template). It has no 5'–3' exonuclease activity. The preparation used for sequencing ("Sequenase") usually has the 3'–5' exonuclease activity inactivated. This was first done chemically, but it is now done by manipulation of the polymerase gene to produce a form of the enzyme called "Sequenase 2.0".

2. RNA-dependent DNA polymerases. These enzymes are also known as *reverse transcriptases*, often abbreviated to RTases, owing to their ability to reverse the usual flow of information by transcription in the "central dogma". They are encoded by retroviruses, which have an RNA genome that has to be turned into DNA as part of their life cycle. (The DNA is subsequently inserted into the host's genome.) A widely used preparation is the product of the *pol* gene of avian myeloblastosis virus (AMV). Like other DNA polymerases, RTases need a primer that is hydrogen-bonded to the template, and they direct DNA synthesis in a 5'–3' direction. In virally infected cells, the primer is a cellular tRNA molecule that shows complementarity to part of the retroviral genome. In the lab, a suitable primer must be supplied. RTases' most important use is in the synthesis of DNA from RNA when making cDNA libraries, as described in Section 4.3.3. They can also be used in sequencing – either in direct sequencing of RNA, provided a suitable primer is available, or in DNA sequencing, since they can use DNA as well as RNA as a template. RTase has no proofreading 3'–5' exonuclease activity and therefore has an error rate higher than that of most polymerases. Under standard conditions the error rate can be as high as 1 incorrectly incorporated nucleotide in 500, and this should be taken into account when using clones obtained with reverse transcriptase (although it often isn't).

3. DNA-dependent RNA polymerases. As well as encoding DNA polymerases, viruses can encode their own RNA polymerases. Because the phage RNA polymerases are very specific to phage promoters, viruses can inactivate the host RNA polymerase while maintaining transcription of their own genomes. That means that more ribonucleotides, amino acids, and so forth, are available for synthesis of viral RNA and proteins. The phage RNA polymerases, such as those from T3, T7, and SP6, are used in conjunction with the appropriate phage promoters to direct high levels of very specific transcription. They can be used *in vivo* or *in vitro*.

1.3.3 Exonucleases

We have already dealt with *endo*nucleases and their role in cutting DNA up into discrete fragments, and also with the use of the *exo*nucleolytic functions of DNA polymerases. Cells also contain exonucleases that do not have any associated polymerase activity and that have a wide range of roles. We can exploit them for the removal of single-stranded ends, which we have already discussed, and also for the shortening of double-stranded DNA. The latter is particularly useful in constructing collections of clones for DNA sequencing (see Section 3.2.3) and also for targeted mutagenesis (see Sections 7.2.1 and 7.3.2). Exonucleolytic shortening of double-stranded DNA can be carried out in two ways (refer to Figure 1.5).

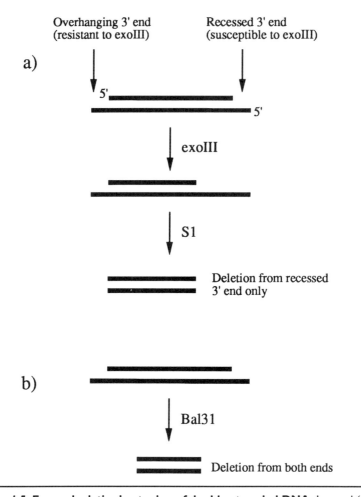

***Figure 1.5* Exonucleolytic shortening of double-stranded DNA.** In panel (**a**), use of exoIII and S1 nuclease leads to deletion from recessed 3' ends (overhanging 5' ends) but not overhanging 3' ends (recessed 5' ends). In panel (**b**), use of Bal31 leads to deletion from both.

1. Removal of strands separately. One technique for shortening double-stranded DNA involves removing one strand at a time. The DNA is linearized (if it is initially circular) by digestion with a restriction enzyme leaving protruding 5' ends. Then it is treated with two separate enzymes. The first is commonly exonuclease III (exoIII). This degrades a single strand of the double-stranded DNA molecule in a 3'–5' direction. It therefore degrades one strand of the duplex at one end and the other strand at the other end, leaving a single-stranded region at each end. The second enzyme used is a single-strand-specific exonuclease (i.e., one that will degrade single-stranded DNA only) such as S1 nuclease from *Aspergillus oryzae* or mung bean nuclease. This polishes up the single-stranded ends left by exoIII.

As described, this technique leads to a molecule's being shortened from both ends, and this is not always desirable. It is possible to protect one end of a molecule from degradation by exploiting the fact that exoIII will not attack *pro-truding* 3' ends (as these are effectively just single-stranded molecules and the enzyme works only on double-stranded ones). The target molecule is cut with two restriction enzymes chosen so that the resulting fragment to be shortened has one protruding 3' end and one recessed end. Subsequent treatment with exoIII degrades only the latter end, which is then polished with S1 or mung bean nuclease.

Protection from exoIII can also be achieved by replacing a nucleotide at one end by a phosphorothioate nucleotide analogue, which is resistant to removal by exoIII. (Incorporation of the analogue can be achieved by end-filling a restriction fragment in the presence of the analogue.)

2. Removal of both strands together. Some exonucleases can remove both strands of a base-paired duplex concurrently. One such is Bal31. Its main activity is a 3'–5' exonuclease, which generates single-stranded ends. These are then degraded by an endonuclease activity that the enzyme also has. Treatment of DNA with Bal31 will therefore lead to simultaneous removal of bases from both strands at both ends, although in practice some overhangs may be left, because the endonuclease lags behind the exonuclease.

In both methods for exonucleolytic shortening, the extent of the deletion will depend on the amounts of nuclease added and the incubation time. Controlling these parameters therefore allows the extent of the deletions to be manipulated. By taking samples from the reaction after different times, one can produce a "nested" series of deletions with a range of lengths.

1. 3. 4 Methylases

We have already seen that the modification side of restriction-modification systems protects a cell's DNA by methylation at the recognition site. Sometimes in cloning it is necessary to protect DNA artificially against cleavage by a particular enzyme, often *Eco*RI (see Section 2.4.1). That can therefore be done by treating the DNA with *Eco*RI methylase, which transfers methyl groups onto the DNA from S-adenosyl methionine.

1. 4 LIGATION

Ligation is the alignment of the ends of two (usually double-stranded) DNA molecules and the formation of a covalent linkage (phosphodiester bond) between them in one or both strands. A break in the sugar-phosphate backbone of a DNA molecule that can be sealed simply by the formation of a phosphodiester bond is called a *nick*. If nucleotides are missing, then it is called a *gap* and cannot be sealed by ligase alone.

1. 4. 1 Categories of reaction

Ligation reactions may be *blunt-ended* or *sticky-ended*. In the former, the molecules to be joined do not have overhanging single-stranded ends, which would have the potential to reanneal. The ends might, for example, have been generated directly by the action of a restriction endonuclease that gives a straight cut or by polishing the ends of molecules produced with an enzyme that generates staggered cuts. In sticky-ended ligation, the molecules have complementary single-stranded ends. The ends can base-pair, and the ligase then forms the phosphodiester bond(s) to seal the nicks. The reaction is most efficient if the sticky ends complement each other exactly. A small amount of mismatch may be acceptable, though. In general, ligation of correctly matched ends is more efficient than ligation of blunt ends. However, the energy required to break the few hydrogen bonds holding sticky ends together is very low – comparable with the vibrational and kinetic energy of molecules at room temperature. Sticky-ended ligations are therefore often done at lower than room temperature, usually at 4°C.

Ligation reactions may be *intermolecular*, in which the end of one molecule is ligated to the end of another, or *intramolecular*, in which the end of one molecule is ligated to the other end of the same molecule, resulting in its circularization. The former requires collision between two separate molecules and implies second order kinetics; the latter implies first order kinetics. Decreasing the volume of a reaction will increase the probability that two separate molecules will collide but will not alter the probability that one end of a molecule will meet the other one. It should therefore enhance the frequency of intermolecular ligations compared to intramolecular ones. The effective volume of a reaction can be decreased by adding a volume excludant such as polyethylene glycol.

1. 4. 2 Ligases

Ligases are part of the routine battery of enzymes required by a cell for the maintenance of its DNA. They are used in joining together adjacent Okazaki fragments produced in replication and are used in sealing the nicks that arise from damage and from repair processes. A deficiency of one of the ligases found in human cells is responsible for Bloom's syndrome, in which replication is slowed and there is greater sensitivity to DNA-damaging agents and a higher susceptibility to cancer. Like the DNA polymerases we discussed earlier, the ligases that we will use can come from normal *E. coli* or cells that have been infected by viruses.

1. **T4 DNA ligase** is encoded by bacteriophage T4, and is produced upon infection of *E. coli* cells. It can carry out both blunt-ended and sticky-ended ligations and requires ATP. It requires a 3'-hydroxyl and a 5'-phosphate group on the molecules to be joined.

2. ***E. coli* DNA ligase** is the endogenous bacterial enzyme. Unlike T4 DNA ligase, it is unable to carry out blunt-ended ligations (or does so only very inefficiently) and is therefore particularly useful if such ligations need to be avoided. This might be the case if one were trying to seal nicks in damaged DNA without also joining noncontiguous sequences. *E. coli* DNA ligase is usually more expensive than T4 DNA ligase, so routine sticky-ended ligations are usually done with the latter. Like the T4 ligase, *E. coli* DNA ligase requires a 3'-hydroxyl and a 5'-phosphate group, but it requires NAD^+ as a cofactor. Essentially the same reaction is catalysed by each of these ligases; this reaction is shown in Figure 1.6. In both cases, AMP is added to the 5'-phosphate, liberating either pyrophosphate from ATP or nicotinamide mononucleotide from NAD^+. The AMP is then displaced in a nucleophilic attack by the 3'-hydroxyl.

That concludes our survey of the enzymes that we will need to use for the techniques discussed in the forthcoming chapters. There are a few techniques that need to be mentioned now before we can really start, because they are par-

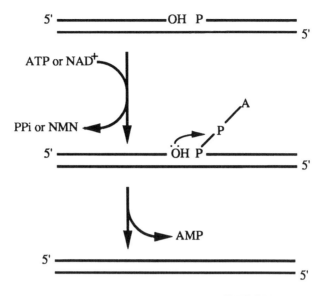

Figure 1.6 **Mechanism of ligation by T4 DNA ligase (using ATP) or *E. coli* ligase (using NAD⁺).**

ticularly relevant. We will consider briefly the extraction of plasmids from *E. coli*, since this operation is one of the most frequent ones in a cloning project. We will also cover gel electrophoresis of nucleic acids, since many general textbooks do not cover all aspects adequately for our purposes, and blotting. We will look briefly at the synthesis of oligonucleotides with defined sequences. DNA sequencing will be covered in a later chapter (Section 3.2.3), since it depends greatly on the application of particular cloning techniques. We will not go into details of the purification of DNA, RNA, or protein from cells other than *E. coli*, since the protocols vary widely from one organism to another, and long lists of practical instructions would not be appropriate here. Nor will we consider general molecular biological techniques, such as transcript mapping and gel retardation assays. Although they can be important in the analysis of cloned genes, they are now quite routine throughout molecular biology, and more general textbooks give details.

1.5 PURIFICATION OF PLASMID DNA FROM *E. COLI*

Probably one of the most frequent operations in cloning work is the preparation of plasmid DNA from *E. coli*. Isolation of genomic DNA from other organisms follows similar principles. There are a number of different techniques, but essentially they involve the same operations:

    a. cell lysis

    b. removal of proteins and chromosomal DNA

    c. collection of plasmid DNA

    d. further purification if necessary

There are many laboratory manuals that provide practical details, so we will settle for a brief outline. Commonly, cells are lysed by treatment with lysozyme (which hydrolyses the N-acetyl glucosamine–N-acetyl muramic acid polypeptide chain of the cell wall) and often also detergents. The chromosomal DNA is removed by centrifugation (because the molecule is so large it can be pelleted by centrifugation in a benchtop microcentrifuge), and the proteins are removed by extraction into phenol and chloroform. The nucleic acid remaining is then precipitated, usually by the addition of sodium or ammonium acetate and ethanol. (Variations on this include the use of boiling, or of sodium hydroxide and sodium dodecyl sulphate to denature the proteins and the chromosomal DNA in order to facilitate their removal by centrifugation. DNA may also be separated by adsorption onto a suitable solid-phase material followed by elution, rather than by precipitation.)

The precipitated nucleic acid includes plasmid DNA, any chromosomal DNA that centrifugation did not remove, and RNA. Chromosomal DNA contamination should be low, and RNA can be destroyed if necessary with ribonuclease, so the precipitated nucleic acids may be suitable for use without further purification. If necessary, caesium chloride density gradient centrifugation can be used. This relies on the fact that a solution of caesium chloride, if spun in an ultracentrifuge, will form a concentration (and density) gradient because the caesium ions are so heavy. The nucleic acids and caesium chloride are dissolved and subjected to centrifugation. The gradient of caesium chloride concentration and density then forms, and the DNA migrates to the position in the gradient where its own density (determined by whether the DNA is supercoiled and by the G+C content – with a higher G+C content giving a greater density) is equal to that of the surrounding solution. This is an equilibrium position, and further centrifugation will not alter the position of the DNA. The closed circular plasmid DNA forms a band at one position in the centrifuge tube. Nicked (and therefore not supercoiled) plasmid DNA and linear fragments of chromosomal DNA form a band higher in the tube. RNA forms a pellet at the bottom of the tube, and any protein left floats to the surface. The location of the plasmid DNA is determined by including the orange-red stain ethidium bromide in the solution before centrifugation. The ethidium bromide molecule is very flat (Figure 1.2) and intercalates between the stacked bases of a piece of double-stranded nucleic acid. Once inserted, it will fluoresce very brightly with a rosy pink colour under ultraviolet (UV) light, because energy is transmitted to it from the DNA itself. The fluorescence can be used to locate the DNA in the centrifuge tube. However, there is often so much ethidium bromide intercalated in the plasmid DNA that UV illumination is not necessary. Once the DNA has been collected, the ethidium bromide is removed by washing it with butanol. Caesium chloride is removed by dialysis, and the DNA is precipitated and redissolved.

1. 6. GEL ELECTROPHORESIS OF NUCLEIC ACIDS

1. 6. 1 The principle

The basic use we will make of gel electrophoresis is to separate nucleic acid molecules by size (although the technique is equally applicable to proteins). In essence, a gel that contains buffer is formed by a meshwork of molecules, and nucleic acids are driven through it by an electric field. At the pHs used, the charge on a DNA molecule results from the negatively charged phosphate groups of the sugar-phosphate backbone. So the charge on the molecule, and therefore the force attracting it to the positive terminal, will be directly proportional to the number of phosphate groups on it and, therefore, to its length. The mass of the molecule will also be proportional to its length (if we ignore the effects caused by the differences in molecular weights of the bases, which are negligible). The force per unit mass on a molecule, and therefore the acceleration towards the anode, will consequently be independent of the size of the molecule. If unhindered, all molecules would therefore move in the electric field at the same speed. However, the gel matrix retards the progress of the molecules, which in effect become entangled in it. Small linear molecules are able to pass through more freely than large ones, and so move faster through the gel. The DNA molecules are therefore separated by size, with smaller ones moving further. Electrophoresis is carried out for a given length of time, and the positions of the DNA are visualized (generally by staining the gel with ethidium bromide or by autoradiography if the DNA is radioactive). Through comparison of the positions with those of standards of known sizes run in the same gel, the sizes of molecules under analysis (e.g., the products of a restriction digest) can be estimated. It is found empirically that for linear molecules, a graph of the distance moved against the logarithm of the size of the fragment gives a straight line over a reasonable range. The behaviour of circular molecules is not as simple, and the retardation by the gel matrix depends on the topological parameters of the molecule (the degree of supercoiling, etc.). Different topological forms can be distinguished by their mobilities, but absolute size estimates are generally unreliable.

1. 6. 2   Gel matrices

Two gel matrices are favoured: agarose and polyacrylamide. Agarose is a purified polysaccharide from rhodophyte ("red") algae of the genera *Gelidium* and *Gracilaria* and is composed of modified galactose residues. (In conjunction with another polysaccharide, agaropectin, it forms agar.) The agarose is dissolved by boiling in buffer and then allowed to cool. This results in the formation of a gel at room temperature. Polyacrylamide is formed by the polymerization of acrylamide and N,N'-methylene-*bis*-acrylamide, which crosslinks the chains. The structures of these three molecules are shown in Figure 1.7. Polymerization is brought about by the addition of ammonium persulphate and tetramethylethylenediamine (TEMED). The TEMED catalyses the formation of free radicals from the persulphate ions, and these initiate polymerization of the acrylamide. Agarose gels are usually cast and run in flat trays, and polyacrylamide gels are usually cast and run vertically between two glass plates. Because of the effective pore sizes in the gel matrices and the concentrations of polyacrylamide and agarose that are convenient to work with, polyacrylamide gels are best suited for electrophoresis of molecules up to 1 kb, and agarose gels are best suited for molecules from a few hundred bases and up. Of course, some variation in the concentrations used is possible to suit the requirements of a given experiment.

   If it is necessary to electrophorese *single-stranded* DNA or RNA, denaturing gels are usually necessary in order to stop complementary strands from reannealing, and intramolecular base-pairing from forming secondary structures, which would affect the mobility. Use of denaturing gels is particularly important in DNA sequencing, in which the ability to resolve molecules differ-a)

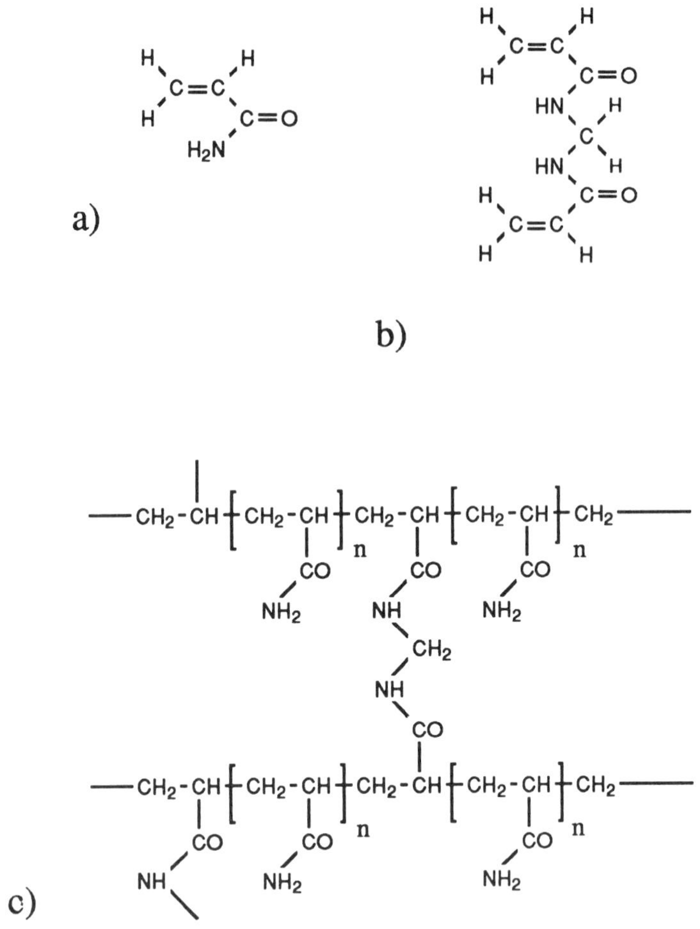

b)

c)

Figure 1.7 **Structures of acrylamide (a), N, N'-methylene-*bis*-acrylamide (b), and polyacrylamide (c).**

ing in length by a single nucleotide is necessary. Denaturing gels can be run using exactly the same matrices that are used with nondenaturing ones, with the addition of denaturing agents. These agents interfere with the formation of secondary structure and include urea, formamide, and formaldehyde. Electrophoresis at elevated temperature (the heating caused by the electric current in the gel may be sufficient) also helps to disrupt secondary structure.

It is often useful to be able to recover material, usually DNA, from gels. Perhaps one needs to clone a specific restriction fragment from a digest by separating the desired fragment from the others using a gel and then recovering it from the gel for cloning. There are several ways of doing this:

1. Diffusion. A slice containing the DNA to be recovered is cut from the gel, crushed, and soaked in buffer for several hours. Most of the DNA diffuses from the gel, which can be removed by filtration or centrifugation.

2. Freeze-squeeze. A slice containing the DNA is cut from the gel and frozen in liquid nitrogen. This breaks up the structure of the gel. It is then centrifuged through a glass wool plug. The plug stops the gel but allows the liquid from it (with dissolved DNA) to pass through.

3. Melting. The melting technique is applicable only to agarose gels with a low gelling temperature. The slice is cut from the gel and melted by warming. The DNA is then recovered by suitable solvent extraction.

4. Electroelution. There are several techniques involving electroelution. Here are three.

> **a.** A slice is cut from the gel, sealed into dialysis tubing containing buffer, and subjected to further electrophoresis. The DNA leaves the gel, but is retained in the buffer in the dialysis tubing.

> **b.** A slot is cut in the gel *adjacent* to and beyond the DNA of interest and filled with buffer, and electrophoresis is continued. The DNA falls out of the gel into the slot containing the buffer, whence it can be removed with a pipette.

> **c.** A piece of a suitable membrane is inserted into the gel adjacent to the DNA and electrophoresis is continued. The DNA sticks to the membrane. The membrane is removed and the DNA washed off with an appropriate solution. One suitable membrane is DEAE-cellulose, from which DNA can be removed by washing with a high-salt buffer.

5. Agarase. The enzyme agarase is used to digest the gel matrix, and the DNA is purified by phenol extraction.

I.6.3 Visualization

There are several ways of visualizing nucleic acids in gels. One of the easiest is to stain the gel with ethidium bromide and use fluorescence under UV light to locate the DNA. A related method is *UV shadowing*. Here the gel is placed on a UV-fluorescent screen. UV light is shone onto the gel and passes through it to the screen, causing the latter to fluoresce. DNA in the gel, however, will absorb the UV light, stopping it from reaching the screen. A nonfluorescing shadow will therefore be seen under regions of the gel that contain DNA. This technique is useful when dealing with single-stranded material, into which ethidium bromide does not intercalate very efficiently. It also has the advantage that it is not necessary subsequently to remove intercalated ethidium bromide, which may be difficult to do completely. Other dyes, such as methylene blue, can be used to locate DNA, although these are less sensitive. Radiolabelled DNA can of course be detected by autoradiography or fluorography.

I.6.4 Field strength gradient gels

A consequence of the way molecules are separated in a gel is that the greatest separation for a given difference in molecule length is obtained amongst the smallest DNA molecules, at the "bottom," or anode, of the gel. Particularly in DNA sequencing, it may be desirable to increase the separation in the upper part of the gel and reduce that in the lower. That can be done by having a nonuniform electric field strength (potential difference per unit length) in the gel, with a weaker field towards the bottom of the gel. The consequence is that as molecules move further in the gel they experience a weaker field and so move more slowly. Molecules at the bottom of the gel therefore get separated less for a given difference in molecular length at the expense of those higher up.

Since the same current must flow through any cross section of the gel, the gradient in field strength can be set up using a gradient in resistance, with lower resistance at the bottom of the gel. That is usually achieved in one of two ways. *Wedge* gels can be used, which are thicker and therefore of lower resistance at the bottom. Alternatively, *buffer gradient* gels can be used, in which the concentration of buffer increases (and therefore resistance decreases) towards the bottom of the gel.

1. 6. 5   Pulsed-field gels

Pulsed-field gel electrophoresis (PFGE) can be used for separating DNA molecules much larger than those suitable for conventional electrophoresis, and can separate whole chromosomes. Very large DNA molecules – those above a certain threshold dictated by the pore size of the gel – can only pass through the matrix by threading through, oriented parallel to the direction of movement. Movement in any direction other than the one in which the molecule is "pointing" is blocked by the gel matrix. Above that threshold size, all DNA molecules (if correctly oriented) will pass at the same speed. The principle of PFGE is to apply alternating electric fields across the gel in pulses, often at 90° to each other, although other angles can be used. Once the field position alters, the large molecules are unable to move until they become reoriented along the direction of the field. This takes longer for larger molecules. Therefore, provided the length of the pulse is greater than the time needed for reorientation, the time available for actual movement through the gel (and consequently the distance moved) will increase as the size of the molecule decreases. It is possible to resolve DNA molecules that are several megabases in size. There are several modifications to the technique – varying, for example, the position of the fields relative to one another, the relative strengths of the fields, and the absolute and relative lengths of the pulses.

1. 6. 6   Blotting

It is often necessary to transfer DNA or RNA from a gel to a membrane as a solid-phase support. This is called *blotting* and can be achieved using the arrangement shown in Figure 1.8. Buffer flows up from the reservoir via a wick, through the gel and the membrane over it, into the stack of paper towels above it. The nucleic acids are carried by the buffer but are trapped by the membrane over the gel. It is possible to assist the transfer electrophoretically or by use of a vacuum. The apparatus is then dismantled and the membrane removed. The nucleic acid can be denatured, if necessary (though it is usually denatured before transfer), and fixed to the membrane by heat treatment or UV crosslinking. If the membrane is then immersed in a solution containing labelled nucleic acids (a *probe)* complementary to some of the sequences on the membrane, the labelled probe will hybridize to the complementary material on the membrane. The position of the bound probe can then be visualized, for example, by autoradiography if the probe is radioactively labelled. The technique, therefore, allows one to work out which regions of a gel contain sequences corresponding to the

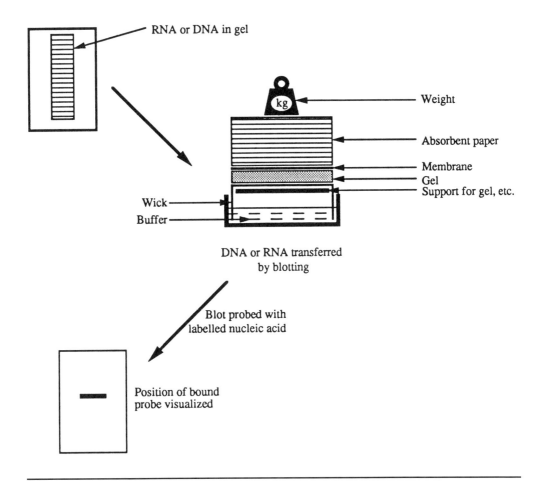

RNA or DNA in gel

Weight

Absorbent paper

Membrane

Gel

Support for gel, etc.

Wick

Buffer

DNA or RNA transferred
by blotting

Blot probed with
labelled nucleic acid

Position of bound
probe visualized

Figure 1.8 **Blotting of a gel.**

probe. So, for example, it can be used to identify which fragment in the products of a restriction digest contains a sequence corresponding to a cloned gene
used as a probe. If the gel contains mRNA, the technique will indicate the size
class of mRNA (estimated by its position in the gel) that corresponds to the
gene probe. A blot made from a gel containing DNA is usually called a
Southern blot, after its inventor, Ed Southern. A *Northern blot* is one taken from
a gel containing RNA. It is possible to avoid transferring the DNA or RNA
from the gel and to probe the gel directly. Sometimes referred to as hybridization *in gello,* this approach is less sensitive than the conventional one. It can be
useful, however, when the nucleic acid molecules in the gel are very large (tens
of kilobases or more), which may reduce the efficiency of their transfer.

1.7 OLIGONUCLEOTIDE SYNTHESIS

Oligonucleotides of defined sequence are used widely, for example, as primers
in DNA sequencing (see Section 3.2.3), or for identifying complementary DNA
molecules by hybridization. They are synthesized chemically by the coupling of

one nucleotide onto another, and although there are various approaches to synthesis, the principle is the same. Synthesis relies on the ability to block selectively the reactive groups on a nucleotide in order to limit the reaction to the addition of one nucleotide at a time. Thus an individual round of coupling will result in the addition of a single nucleotide. Unblocking one of the reactive groups then allows the addition of another nucleotide, and so on. Mixtures of nucleotides can be used in any round to allow the synthesis of a mixed population, in which different molecules can have different nucleotides at the corresponding position. Clearly, this technique is very repetitive, lending itself to automation, and a large variety of machines for it are now available.

CHAPTER

2

Simple Cloning

2.1 THE BASIC EXPERIMENT

Now that we have surveyed the enzymes and techniques that are used in cloning, we can take an easy example and see how they are applied. One of the simplest exercises is inserting DNA into *E. coli* in a plasmid such as pBR322 (Figure 2.1). Bacterial plasmids are circular double-stranded DNA molecules capable of replicating in bacterial cells. The pBR322 plasmid is rarely used for cloning nowadays, as it is such a simple one; however, its simplicity makes it a helpful example to start with, and many more advanced plasmids include parts of it. It carries two genes of particular importance. One confers resistance to the antibiotic ampicillin, which blocks the crosslinking of the polysaccharide chains in the bacterial cell walls. The lack of crosslinking weakens the bacterial wall, and the cells eventually lyse. The resistance gene encodes an enzyme, called a beta-lactamase, that hydrolyses the beta-lactam ring of the antibiotic and inactivates it. The other gene confers resistance to tetracycline, an antibiotic that inhibits protein synthesis. The resistance gene encodes an enzyme that acetylates the tetracycline and thus inactivates it. The structures of these antibiotics are shown in Figure 2.2. As well as these antibiotic resistance genes, the plasmid has some less immediately obvious features that we will look at in more detail later, such as an origin of replication. It also has a number of recognition

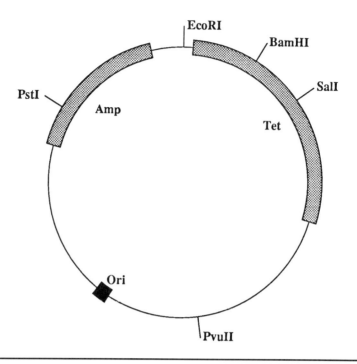

Figure 2.1 **The plasmid pBR322 (4.3 kb),** showing genes for ampicillin resistance (Amp), tetracycline resistance (Tet), the origin of replication (Ori), and selected unique restriction sites.

sites for restriction endonucleases, and some of these are located within the ampicillin and tetracycline resistance genes. These are also shown in Figure 2.1. Suppose we want to clone DNA from the organism we were studying into, say, the *Bam*HI site of pBR322, which is located in the tetracycline resistance gene. (We don't have to use the *Bam*HI site. We could use any of the other restriction sites in either of the genes.) The procedure would be as follows.

The first stage is to purify genomic DNA from the organism of interest and cut it with the enzyme *Bam*HI. We would also purify some pBR322 and cut it with the same enzyme. Then the *Bam*HI-digested plasmid and the *Bam*HI-digested genomic DNA are mixed, and DNA ligase in a suitable buffer is added. *Bam*HI ends will anneal to *Bam*HI ends, and the ligase will seal the nicks. That will generate a large number of types of molecule, shown in Figure 2.3. Intramolecular ligation of plasmid DNA will regenerate the original circular pBR322 plasmid (*a* in Figure 2.3). Intramolecular ligation of genomic DNA will produce circular molecules of genomic DNA (*b*), with no plasmid DNA sequences present. A wide range of intermolecular ligations can take place. Two plasmid DNA molecules can be ligated, in either a head-to-head (*c*) or head-to-tail (*d*) configuration. Two genomic DNA molecules can be ligated, again in either orientation (*e*). Most important, a genomic DNA molecule can be ligated to a plasmid DNA molecule (*f*). (Of course, a huge range of ligations involving three or more molecules can also take place, but they will be rarer than unimolecular or bimolecular ones. How rare depends on the concentrations of the

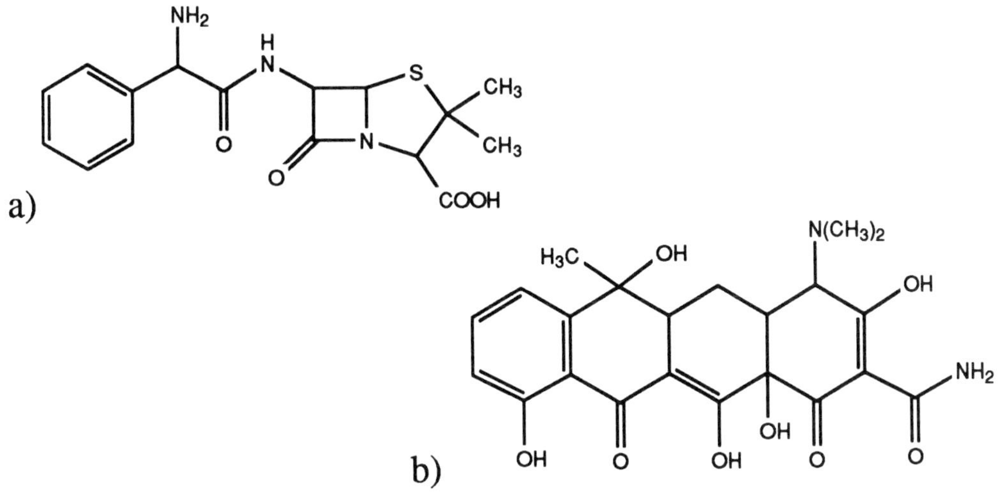

Figure 2.2 **Structures of ampicillin (a) and tetracycline (b).**

species involved.) The molecules that contain new combinations of sequences, not present before, are termed *recombinants*. Note that the insertion of DNA into the tetracycline resistance gene will destroy the function of that gene, and it is therefore an easy matter to work out what properties each of the plasmid types shown in Figure 2.3 will confer. (It is possible that insertion of a short piece of DNA into the tetracycline resistance gene might not inactivate the gene function, if the reading frame were not terminated or shifted. This is relatively rare, but the possibility should always be kept in mind.)

The next stage is to put the ligation products back into *E. coli*. That is a process called *transformation,* and we will deal with the details of it in a moment. An important point is that transformation is rather inefficient, in that the probability of any individual bacterial cell's taking up a piece of DNA is very low. For simple transformation procedures, of 10^9 cells treated with 1 microgram of supercoiled plasmid DNA, typically only 10^5 or so will successfully take up a molecule. We say there is a *transformation frequency* of 10^5 colonies/microgram of DNA. This is low, given that 1 microgram of pBR322 contains of the order of 10^{11} molecules. Because the probability of a cell's taking up one DNA molecule is low, the probability of its taking up two is very low indeed. (Actually, that need not be the case. It could be that only a tiny proportion of cells are able to take up DNA, but those that do are very efficient at it and will take up more than one piece. In fact, it does seem that very few cells take up more than one piece. It may be true that only a fraction of the cells are able to take up DNA, but they still do so very inefficiently.) The cells are now plated on agar containing, in this example, ampicillin. The cells that did not take up a plasmid will be sensitive to the antibiotic and die after a few generations. Those that took up genomic DNA only – *b* and *e* in Figure 2.3 – will also die. Those that took up pBR322 DNA – *a, c, d,* and *f* – will have acquired an ampicillin resistance gene and will be able to grow on the selective medium. They will therefore form isolated colonies on the agar if plated at a suitable dilution. All the members of a colony are derived from one

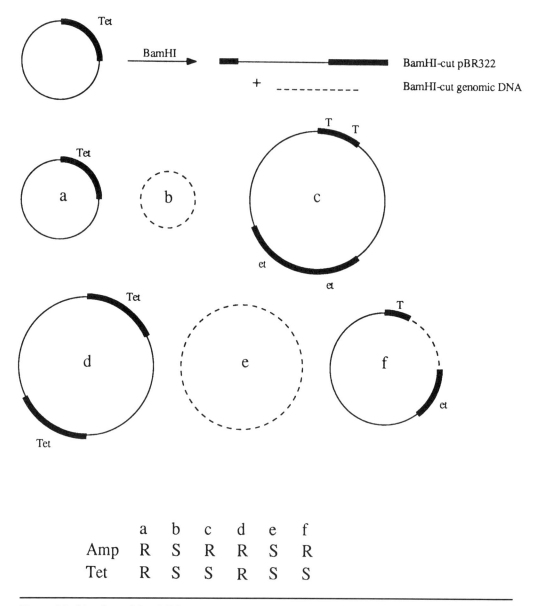

	a	b	c	d	e	f
Amp	R	S	R	R	S	R
Tet	R	S	S	R	S	S

Figure 2.3 Ligation of *Bam*HI fragments (dashed) into *Bam*HI-cut pBR322 DNA. The tetracy-cline resistance gene is shown by the heavy line. **T** and **et** indicate the parts of the gene before and after the *Bam*HI site. The labelled circles show the results of religation of the plasmid (**a**), self-ligation of a single piece of genomic DNA (**b**), head-to-head ligation of two plasmid molecules (**c**), head-to-tail ligation of two plasmid molecules (**d**), ligation of two genomic DNA fragments (**e**), and ligation of a vector molecule and a genomic DNA fragment (**f**). **R** indicates that the molecule confers resistance to ampicillin or tetracycline, **S** that it does not.

cell and should therefore have acquired a single plasmid. (If a cell did manage to acquire more than one plasmid, the colony would have a mixture and the subsequent analysis would be much more complicated.)

The problem now is to distinguish the colonies that have acquired genomic DNA (*f*) from all the others. That can be done in this example by taking a sample of each colony and plating it onto tetracycline. The ones that have acquired type *a* or type *d* molecules will have an intact tetracycline resistance gene. Those that have acquired type *c* or type *f* molecules will be killed by the tetracycline (which is why it is important to use only a sample from each ampicillin-resistant colony, and not the whole thing). The relative abundances of type *c* and type *f* molecules will depend on the relative proportions of genomic and plasmid DNA in the initial ligation. The molecules can be differentiated by growing up colonies, purifying plasmid DNA, and cutting it with a restriction enzyme. *Bam*HI would be the easiest in this case and would generate two sizes of molecule in type *f* – plasmid DNA and genomic DNA – but a single size in type *c*

The outcome of this experiment is a large number of *E. coli* colonies, each carrying a plasmid containing a *Bam*HI fragment of genomic DNA. That is useful in a number of ways. For example, to get a lot more of each piece of genomic DNA, it is just a matter of growing up a larger quantity of *E. coli*, extracting the plasmid, and if necessary, separating the insert from the plasmid. That is much easier than extracting the DNA from more of the organism(s) we used in the first place. Also, each plasmid insert is a single, defined piece of DNA. To separate a single, defined piece out of the total genomic DNA each time one wanted it would be too laborious. This is *cloning* – the propagation of individual, defined pieces of DNA in a suitable organism.

The generation of recombinants in this way – randomly cloning fragments of the total DNA from an organism – is called *shotgun* cloning, and the random collection of *E. coli* colonies containing the recombinant DNA molecules is called a *library*. Because total genomic DNA was used, it is called a *genomic library*. An ideal genomic library would contain all the sequences present in the original organism's genome and would then be described as *representative*. A library constructed in the way we have just described would probably not be very representative. For example, small DNA fragments tend to be cloned more efficiently than large ones, so our library would be underrepresentative of the large fragments. Another problem with the library in our example is that any gene that contained a *Bam*HI site could never be rescued intact, because *Bam*HI digestion was used to generate the fragments to be cloned. It would be better to use some other way of generating the fragments (see Section 1.2). Now we will go back to the basic procedure we have described and look in a little more detail at some of the steps involved.

2.2. VECTORS, TRANSFORMATION, AND HOSTS

2.2.1 Vectors

Vector is the name given to DNA molecules into which foreign DNA is inserted for subsequent propagation in a host cell. A vector should have several features:

1. An origin of replication. Without an origin of replication, the vector cannot replicate, and when the cells divide after taking up the vector molecule, only one of the daughter cells would retain it. We could therefore never get a colony of transformed cells. The pBR322 origin of replication came from a plasmid in a clinical bacterial isolate denoted as pMB1.

2. A selectable marker. This is needed to distinguish cells that have taken up the vector from those that have not. In the example we have just looked at, the selectable marker was ampicillin resistance. The tetracycline resistance gene of pBR322 could have been used as a selectable marker if a cloning site elsewhere had been used. The ampicillin resistance gene of pBR322 derives from a *transposon* (a piece of DNA able to move, or transpose, to different places in the genome) from another plasmid, pRSF2124, and the tetracycline resistance gene from the plasmid pSC101.

3. Suitable single restriction sites. In the example we considered, pBR322 had just one recognition site for the enzyme *Bam*HI, which was used in the cloning. Had there been more than one *Bam*HI site, then pBR322 would not have been suitable, because cutting with *Bam*HI would have cut the vector into more than one piece. Reassembly of the vector together with an insert during the ligation would have required a trimolecular reaction at least, which would have been very unlikely. Note, though, that the same enzyme does not necessarily have to be used for cutting both vector and insert (see Section 1.2.1). If the insert molecules had been generated by *Sau*3A digestion, we could still have used *Bam*HI to cut the vector, as *Bam*HI ends are compatible with *Sau*3A ends. Cutting the vector with *Sau*3A would not have been feasible, as there are too many sites (22 in pBR322). Note that restriction sites located in indispensable genes are unsuitable for cloning, because insertion of DNA in such genes would be likely to destroy their function and therefore vector viability. We will see that this is particularly important when we consider vectors based on bacterial viruses (Sections 3.2.2 and 3.3.2).

4. Suitable size. To some extent, having a suitable size is a corollary of having suitable single restriction sites. A 6-nucleotide-restriction-enzyme cleavage site will occur on average approximately once every 4^6 bp (i.e., every 4 kb or so). So a vector that was much larger than that might be expected to have several sites for a given enzyme, and cutting the vector would reduce it into several pieces that would be unlikely to be correctly assembled in a ligation reaction. It is possible to remove restriction sites, though, and methods for doing this are described in Section 7.2.1. Simply removing excess restriction sites may not eliminate the problem, though; large DNA molecules are very susceptible to physical shearing – even in the simple act of pipetting – so they are always difficult to handle.

5. Markers for DNA insertion. In the example we studied, the insertion of DNA into the vector can be detected by inactivation of the tetracycline resistance gene, and the inactivation can easily be assayed by plating cells onto a medium containing tetracycline. If the cloning site used had not been in any functional sequence, that approach would not be possible, and the only way to detect insertion would be to isolate plasmid DNAs, digest with a suitable enzyme, and electrophoretically examine the fragments produced. Although that is possible, it would be very tedious, especially if intramolecular ligation had been favoured over the intermolecular reactions (the tendency for which will depend on the relative concentrations of plasmid DNA and genomic DNA), in which case most of the plasmids in transformed cells would not be recombinant.

6. High copy number. Having a high copy number is desirable but not essential, like having markers for DNA insertion. To maximize the yield of plasmid from transformed cells, the copy number in each cell should be as high as possible. Different plasmids have different copy numbers. For some, such as the F factor, the copy number is low – perhaps 1 or 2 per cell. The replication of the F factor is quite closely tied to replication of the chromosome, and such control of replication is said to be *stringent*. The plasmid pSC101 (one of the first plasmids used for this work) is also under stringent control and is usually present at no more than 5 copies per cell. Other plasmids with different origins of replication have less tightly controlled replication, and they are said to be *relaxed*. Here the copy number can range widely. The copy number of pBR322 is typically 15–20 per cell, whereas other vectors, such as the pUC plasmids (see Section 2.3.2), may be present in 500–700 copies per cell. The origin of replication for pBR322 and the pUC plasmids came ultimately from the plasmid pMB1. The reason for the difference in copy number between these plasmids with, in theory, the same replication origin may lie in a mutation in the pUC plasmids in the region encoding the RNA molecules that regulate replication by interacting with the origin. This mutation makes the repression system that controls plasmid replication less effective. The copy number of many low-copy-number plasmids containing the pMB1 origin can be increased by *chloramphenicol amplification*. The host cell culture is treated with chloramphenicol, which inhibits bacterial protein synthesis. The inhibition of protein synthesis blocks chromosomal DNA replication, because particular proteins, such as DnaA, need to be synthesized each time chromosomal replication is initiated. The inhibition also blocks cell division, which is closely tied to chromosomal DNA replication. Plasmid replication, however, only requires enzymes that are more long-lived. It can therefore continue while chromosomal DNA replication and cell division have stopped. Eventually, plasmid DNA replication will stop, too, as the supply of general replication proteins, such as DNA polymerase, runs out, but the average copy number will have increased greatly.

7. Disablement. Ever since the earliest experiments in genetic manipulation, there has been concern over the possibility of recombinant DNA molecules' "escaping" into the environment and spreading. The likelihood of this can be reduced if the plasmid is in some way *disabled* so that it cannot spread by processes such as conjugation. Many plasmids, such as pBR322, have been disabled by removal of the *mob* gene, which is required by them to mobilize themselves by conjugation. However, such plasmids can still be transmitted from cells containing other plasmids that can provide the necessary proteins for mobilization. This transmission can be blocked by removing a region containing sites called *nic* and *bom* from the plasmid that might be mobilized. This region is where the proteins provided by the other plasmids act. The pUC series are among the vectors that have had this region removed.

2. 2. 2 Transformation

Transformation is the direct uptake of naked DNA by cells. In some bacterial species, transformation is an important natural process for increasing genetic variation. The ability to take up naked DNA is called *competence*; it often occurs at a particular stage in the growth of a culture (e.g., stationary phase) and may be associated with the induction of the synthesis of a set of proteins termed *competence proteins*. The degree of competence that is needed experimentally for *E. coli* has to be induced artificially and can be achieved most conveniently in two ways. One involves chemical treatment, the other electric shocks. There are also less simple ways of introducing DNA into bacterial cells. These include the two natural processes of conjugation and phage infection, as well as *biolistic* transformation – the firing of tiny DNA-coated projectiles into the target cells (see Sections 3.2.2, 3.3.2, and 9.6.4).

1. **Chemical induction of competence** classically involves treatment with low temperatures (incubation on ice) and nonphysiological concentrations of divalent cations, followed by brief heat shock. Exactly why this induces the uptake of naked DNA is far from clear. In its simplest form, this approach involves treatment with calcium chloride at concentrations of 30–100 mM, but more complex transformation buffers include manganese chloride and magnesium chloride. Such protocols can generate up to 10^9 transformants per microgram of pBR322, with up to 5% of viable cells competent for transformation. Other treatments have also been used, in attempts to increase the transformation frequency further, and one is often called the *Hanahan* transformation, after its inventor. This involves treatment of the cells with a complex mixture containing KCl, $MnCl_2$, $CaCl_2$, hexamine cobalt trichloride, dimethyl sulphoxide, and dithiothreitol. Other, quicker methods are also available (for example, treatment with polyethylene glycol and dimethyl sulphoxide), but these give a lower proportion of competent cells.

Exactly which protocol will be used depends very much on the particular circumstances. If the number of recombinant molecules available is very small and as many different members of the collection as possible need to be recovered (e.g., in cDNA cloning; see Section 4.3.1), then an efficient system is clearly required. However, if the recombinant molecules are abundant or if they are of just one sort or a few sorts – as when reintroducing a plasmid DNA stock into cells to prepare more of the same plasmid – then one of the quicker, less efficient methods will be quite adequate. If the host strain has not been characterized before, then trial and error may be necessary to determine the most appropriate conditions.

Competent cells can be deep-frozen for future use with relatively little loss of viability or competence (and they are available commercially), so this can also reduce the amount of labour involved.

2. **Electric shock,** in the form of treatment with high voltage electric pulses, can also be used to cause DNA uptake. This procedure, called *electroporation,* probably brings about depolarization of the membrane and the formation of pores in it through which DNA (and other macromolecules) can pass. However, cell contents can be lost, and a balance has to be struck between the uptake of DNA and cell death. When optimized, this approach can yield a higher number of transformants per microgram of DNA than the number yielded by any of the chemical treatments (up to 5×10^{10} per microgram have been claimed for electroporation). The pulse is usually obtained by charging a capacitor and then allowing it to discharge through two electrodes in the bacterial suspension. The parameters to be altered are the field strength of the shock (the maximum potential difference divided by the separation between the electrodes) and the rate of

decay of the voltage. This will be exponential and is determined by the product of the resistance of the total circuit and the capacitance. Typically, a field strength of the order of 15 kV/cm is used, with a decay time constant of about 5 msec. These will usually result in most of the cells remaining viable.

2. 2. 3 Hosts

The *host* is the cell in which the recombinant molecules are to be propagated. Choosing the right host is as important as choosing the right vector. Essential or desirable characters include the following:

1. Efficient transformation. This depends on two main features. One is the ability actually to take DNA into the cell, and this process is very poorly understood. Different genotypes respond differently to the different transformation systems described in Section 2.2.2. Some mutations appear to enhance the efficiency of transformation itself. These include the *deoR* mutation, which seems to assist particularly in the uptake of larger DNA molecules.

The other feature is the presence or absence of endogenous DNA-degrading systems. Many hosts used for cloning are derived from *E. coli* strain K, which contains the K restriction-modification system encoded by the *hsdRMS* locus (see Section 1.2.1). The endonuclease is the product of the *hsdR* gene, and cleaves DNA containing the sequence -AACNNNNNNGTGC-, unless the second of the two adenine residues, and the adenine residue on the other strand opposite the thymine, are methylated. Many hosts therefore have an *hsdR⁻* mutation (or a larger deletion) to avoid cleavage of incoming nonprotected DNA. The *hsdM* gene encodes the methylase that protects against degradation, so passaging through an *hsdR⁻M⁺* strain can be used to allow methylation when it will be subsequently necessary to propagate in an *hsdR⁺* strain.

There are other proteins in *E. coli* strain K that will degrade incoming DNA if it *is* methylated, belonging to the MDRS or methylation-dependent restriction systems. These systems are not as well understood as the Classes I–III restriction-modification systems; they include the endonucleases that are the products of the *mcr* and *mrr* loci, which will degrade DNA containing methylcytosine or methyladenine respectively. Using strains mutant in these loci is therefore desirable, particularly when cloning highly methylated DNA.

The extent of methylation of DNA in the host may also affect the efficiency with which other restriction enzymes will subsequently cleave the DNA *in vitro*. Methylation can be carried out by HsdM, and also by the products of the *dam* and *dcm* genes. The Dam protein methylates adenines at the sequence -GATC-, and Dcm methylates cytosines at the sequences -CCAGG- and -CCTGG-. Some frequently used restriction enzymes have recognition sites that overlap with these and are inhibited by methylation, so DNA prepared from strains that are wild-type for these loci will not be efficiently restricted. Use of *dam⁻* or *dcm⁻* strains has the disadvantage, however, that they are mutagenic. This is because newly replicated double-stranded DNA is hemimethylated (before the methylases reach the newly synthesized material). If the polymerase introduces any errors during synthesis, they will result in a mismatch; these mismatches are normally resolved in the cell by correction to the *methylated* strand. In a *dam⁻* or similar strain, neither strand is methylated, and the mismatch correction is as likely to be to the incorrect (newly synthesized) strand as to the correct one.

2. **Stable maintenance of plasmid.** Once a recombinant has entered the cell – assuming it has escaped any endogenous restriction enzyme activity, has a suitable origin of replication, and so on – it is still not guaranteed a long and comfortable existence. Rearrangement of the recombinant may occur, and the most frequent manifestation of this is partial deletion (i.e., loss of part of the molecule.) This usually occurs by recombination across directly repeated sequences, as shown in Figure 2.4. Not all the plasmid molecules in one cell need undergo the same recombination at the same time, so a heterogeneous population of (in this case) three types of molecule will result: the original, unrecombined one; and the two smaller recombination products, one of which will lack an origin of replication and be lost from the population. The other will still be able to replicate, and it will do so faster than the original molecule because it is smaller. Over a number of rounds of replication, even a small difference in the time required for replication can result in a large difference in the number of molecules present. Generating 1 microgram of DNA from a single copy of a 4-kb plasmid takes about 40 cycles of replication. A plasmid that could replicate 10% faster would, over this period, generate approximately 16 times as much DNA and therefore be by far the most abundant molecule in the preparation. The problem will be exacerbated if the original plasmid is deleterious to the host, perhaps by expression of a protein that is toxic to the cell, and the partial dele-

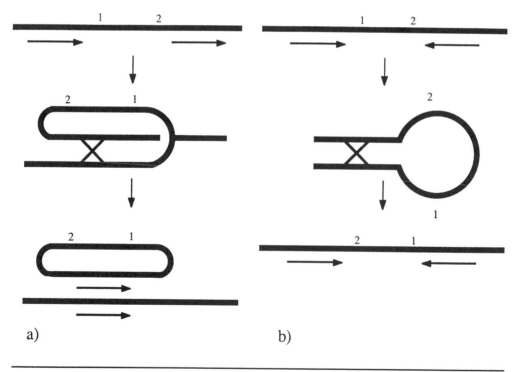

a)   b)

Figure 2.4 **Recombination across repeated sequences.** If the repeats are in a direct configuration, the material between them is lost (**a**). If they are inverted, the material between them is inverted on recombination (**b**). **1** and **2** represent arbitrary points on the molecule.

tion by recombination abolishes production of that protein. The possibility of preferential propagation of altered molecules during cloning is one that should always be borne in mind. Recombination need not always result in deletion. It can also cause inversion, if it takes place across inverted repeats (Figure 2.4).

Since deletions and inversions usually depend upon recombination, mutations in the host that suppress recombination will help to ensure the stability of transforming molecules. There are three main recombination systems in *E. coli*, using the products of the *recBCD, recE,* and *recF* genes. However, all these systems depend largely on the product of the *recA* gene, so strains mutant in this will have a greatly reduced recombination frequency. It seems, however, that some sequences, particularly those containing inverted repeats, may be subject to recombination in a *recA*-independent way. This may be due to the *recF* pathway's functioning in the absence (or at low levels) of *recA*, so a *recF* mutation may be desirable. It is also reported that deficiency of the DNA gyrase encoded by the *gyrA* and *gyrB* genes can lead to enhanced stability of molecules containing repeated sequences.

3. Disablement. As with vectors, it is sensible to take precautions to ensure that strains carrying recombinant plasmids are unlikely to escape and propagate outside the laboratory. For this reason, the preferred strains usually carry a number of mutations to reduce their viability in the wild. These are usually mutations conferring *auxotrophy* (a requirement by the host strain for a particular metabolite to be supplied in the medium, usually resulting from the strain's inability to synthesize it.)

4. Other markers. In any work with bacteria, it is very useful to have strains that are genetically marked, so the correct strains can be recognized as such. The recombination and nutritional deficiency markers mentioned earlier may be useful in this respect, although it may also be convenient to have other markers that can be selected more easily. Antibiotic resistance can be useful, although of course it should be different from any of the antibiotic resistances conferred by the vectors to be used.

Now that we have looked at the basic requirements for a simple cloning experiment, we can look at ways to make the process more efficient or more widely applicable.

2. 3   MODIFICATIONS

One of the most time-consuming aspects of the procedure presented in Section 2.1 is screening the transformants to identify which contain recombinant molecules and which contain religated vector without any insert. There are two particularly important ways of reducing this problem. One is to try to stop it from occurring in the first place. Manipulation of the ratio of vector to insert DNA will go some way towards accomplishing this, although a more reliable solution is to use alkaline phosphatase. The other strategy is to incorporate the selection for inactivation of the gene containing the cloning site into the selection for vector acquisition. This can be done using a somewhat more sophisticated host–vector system.

2. 3. 1   Alkaline phosphatase

Alkaline phosphatase (see Section 1.3.1) is capable of removing 5'-terminal phosphate groups from nucleic acid molecules (and nucleotides). However, these phosphate groups are required for ligation to take place (Section 1.4.2). So if the vector is treated with calf intestinal or shrimp alkaline phosphatase to remove its terminal phosphate groups, self-ligation is no longer possible. Ligation of vector to insert, however, is still possible, because each insert molecule carries two phosphate groups – one at each end. Note though, that sealing each vector–insert boundary requires two phosphate groups – one for each strand. Phosphatase treatment of the vector therefore means that each boundary can be covalently sealed by ligase on one strand only; the other strand will remain nicked, as shown in Figure 2.5. However, these nicks are not a serious problem. Transformation is still possible, and the normal cellular replication and repair processes will produce molecules that are no longer nicked.

In practical terms, the alkaline phosphatase treatment is carried out after the vector has been cut and before vector and insert DNA are mixed. All traces of

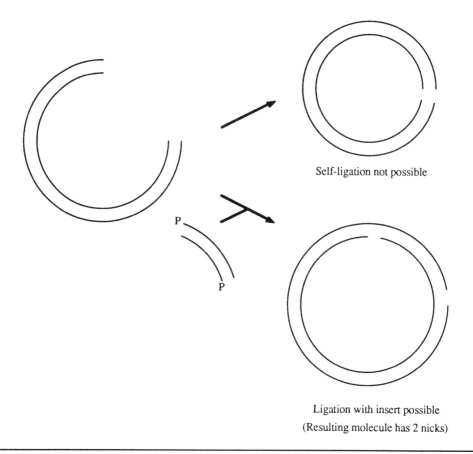

Self-ligation not possible

Ligation with insert possible
(Resulting molecule has 2 nicks)

Figure 2.5 **Phosphatase treatment of vector.** Removal of the phosphate groups (P) from the vector means that self-ligation is not possible. Ligation to a molecule with 5'-phosphates is still possible, although one strand will still be nicked at each junction.

phosphatase activity must be removed before the insert DNA is added; otherwise the insert will be dephosphorylated, too, and intermolecular ligation will also be blocked. One reason for using calf intestinal alkaline phosphatase is that this particular enzyme can readily be inactivated by heating to 75°C for a few minutes. This treatment is usually followed by removal of protein with phenol and chloroform to minimize any carry-over of active enzyme into the ligation reactions. The shrimp enzyme is even more heat labile, and phenol and chloroform purification of the DNA prior to ligation is often omitted.

2.3.2 Amalgamating both rounds of selection: the pUC vectors

Amalgamating both rounds of selection relies on the cloning site used for insertion of DNA being in a gene whose function can be assayed on the same plate as that used for selection of plasmid uptake. The approach often makes use of the *lacZ* gene, which encodes the enzyme beta-galactosidase. This enzyme normally cleaves disaccharides, such as lactose, into monosaccharides, but it can also cleave the artificial substrate 5-bromo-4-chloro-3-indolyl-ß-D-galactoside (also known as X-Gal), shown in Figure 2.6, to liberate a blue dye. For this reason, the substrate is said to be *chromogenic*. It is possible to screen for the production of active beta-galactosidase in bacteria on a plate by including X-Gal and an *inducer* of the *lacZ* gene (i.e., something that activates the gene's expression) in the plate. Usually the gratuitous inducer isopropyl-ß-D-thio-galactoside (IPTG, Figure 2.7) is used. (The term *gratuitous* means that although IPTG acti-

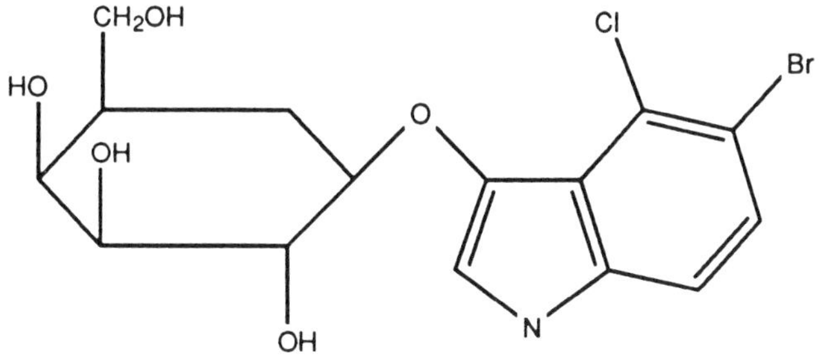

Figure 2.6 **X-Gal (5-bromo-4-chloro-3-indolyl-ß-D-galactoside).**

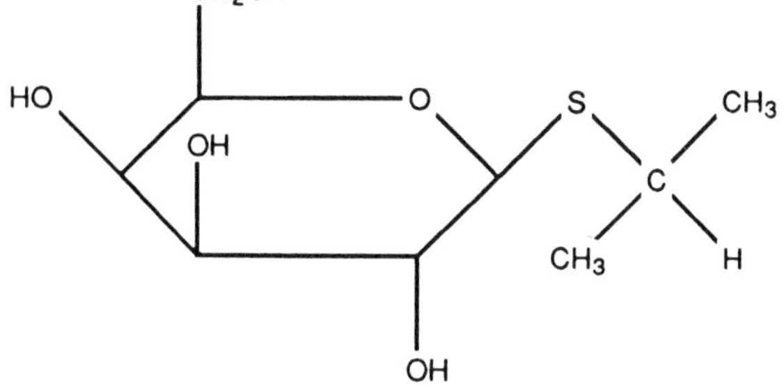

Figure 2.7 **IPTG (isopropyl-ß-D-thio-galactoside).**

vates the *lacZ* gene, the enzyme produced does not degrade it.) Colonies that have a functional *lacZ* gene will be blue, because the chromogenic substrate is cleaved and the blue pigment is produced. Colonies lacking the enzyme will be the normal off-white colour of *E. coli*.

So one could exploit this chromogenic reaction by constructing a plasmid carrying the complete *lacZ* gene and an ampicillin resistance gene, with cloning sites in the *lacZ* gene, and using a host with a mutant *lacZ*. Uptake of plasmid would be selected by ampicillin resistance. Colonies containing plasmid with no insert would be *lacZ*$^+$ and therefore blue. Colonies containing plasmid with an insert disrupting the *lacZ* gene would be *lacZ*$^-$ and therefore white. However, beta-galactosidase is a rather large protein (116 kDa), and it is more convenient to have just a portion of its gene on the vector to keep the latter's size down. The portion used encodes the first 146 amino acids and is called the *minigene*. So the cloning vector contains the ampicillin resistance gene and part of the *lacZ* gene (denoted *lacZ'*), with the cloning sites located in the latter. Many examples of the vectors also contain a *lacI* gene for the Lac repressor, which keeps the minigene repressed except in the presence of an inducer, such as IPTG. (This may be particularly important if the sequences inserted into the minigene are toxic when expressed at high levels.) The rest of the *lacZ* gene is contained on an F' plasmid within the host. In fact, it is a version of the gene called the M15 deletion, which lacks codons 11–41. The polypeptide produced fails to tetramerize, and this tetramerization is needed for enzymatic activity. However, in the presence of the minigene product (amino acids 1–146) assembly can take place to produce an enzyme with low, but detectable, activity. This intragenic complementation is called *alpha-complementation*. This approach, using the *lacZ'* minigene, is exploited by the widely used pUC series of vectors, developed at the University of California (hence their name). It is summarized in Table 2.1 and Figure 2.8.

Clearly, the host must retain the F' plasmid for the system to work. For this reason, the F' plasmid also contains genes *proA* and *proB* for two of the enzymes of proline biosynthesis (encoding gamma-glutamyl phosphate reduc-

---

TABLE 2.1 Alpha-complementation

	LacZ RESIDUES 1–146 PRESENT?	M15-DELETED LacZ PRESENT?	RESULT (+IPTG + X-Gal + Amp)?
Host	No	No	Amp^S, no LacZ; no colonies
Host + F'	No	Yes	Amp^S, no LacZ; no colonies
Host + F' + pUC plasmid	Yes	Yes	Amp^R, LacZ; blue colonies
Host + F' + pUC plasmid (with insert)	No	Yes	Amp^R, no LacZ; white colonies

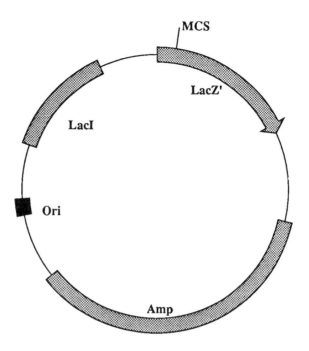

Figure 2.8 **Generalized pUC plasmid**. It contains an ampicillin resistance gene (Amp), part of a beta-galactosidase gene (LacZ'), the Lac repressor gene (LacI), and an origin of replication (Ori). The multiple cloning site (MCS) is located in the beta galactosidase gene.

tase and gamma-glutamyl kinase, respectively), and these are deleted from the chromosome of the host. Propagation of the host on medium lacking proline ensures that only cells carrying the resident F' plasmid will grow. A typical genotype of a host used for pUC plasmids or similar vectors would be that of strain TG2: *supE hsdΔ5 thi* Δ(*lac-proAB*) Δ(*srl-recA*)306::Tn10 F'[*traD36 proAB+lacI*q *lacZΔM15*]. It is worth looking at this genotype in more detail.

supE is an "amber" chain termination suppressor mutation that allows insertion of glutamine residues at UAG codons in translation. It is included because the host is also used for propagation of M13 phages (see Section 3.2.2), and a number of these phages have amber chain termination mutations as a biological containment measure (i.e., one that restricts the ability of recombinant molecules to replicate outside a controlled laboratory situation).

hsdΔ5 inactivates the host K restriction system (see Section 2.2.3).

thi is a nutritional requirement (for thiamine) that gives some containment.

Δ(*lac-proAB*) is the deletion of chromosomal *lac* genes, and *proA* and *proB*, giving a *lac-* host background and allowing selection for the retention of the F' plasmid.

Δ(*srl-recA*)::Tn10 is a transposon-induced inactivation of recombination (see Section 2.2.3).

F' indicates that the genes enclosed in brackets are present on the F' plasmid.

traD36 reduces the efficiency of conjugation by a factor of 10^5, contributing to biological containment.

***proAB*⁺** allows selection for the presence of F' by growth on a medium lacking proline, as previously described.

***lacI*^{q}** is a mutant form of the Lac repressor gene, causing increased levels of repressor in the cell and allowing tighter control of the *lacZ* gene. This is important for the use of this host for vectors that replicate to a high copy number. Such vectors might titrate out all the repressor produced by a wild-type *lacI* gene, especially if the gene was present only on the chromosome or on a low-copy-number plasmid such as F'. Titration of the repressor might lead to uncontrolled transcription of sequences inserted within the *lacZ* region of the vector.

***lacZ*ΔM15** is the partially deleted *lacZ* needed for alpha-complementation.

What about the cloning sites within the *lacZ* minigene? Rather than rely on restriction sites that occurred by chance in the sequence, synthetic DNA was introduced into an *Eco*RI site engineered close to the beginning of the minigene coding region. This DNA was specially designed to have a number of restriction sites within it and is therefore called the *multiple cloning site*. (Sometimes it is called the *polylinker*.) In fact, there is a series of pUC vectors that are differentiated primarily on the sequence at the multiple cloning site. Examples of the cloning sites of two members of this series are given in Figure 2.9. In the earlier constructs, such as pUC7, the multiple cloning site contained pairs of sites for

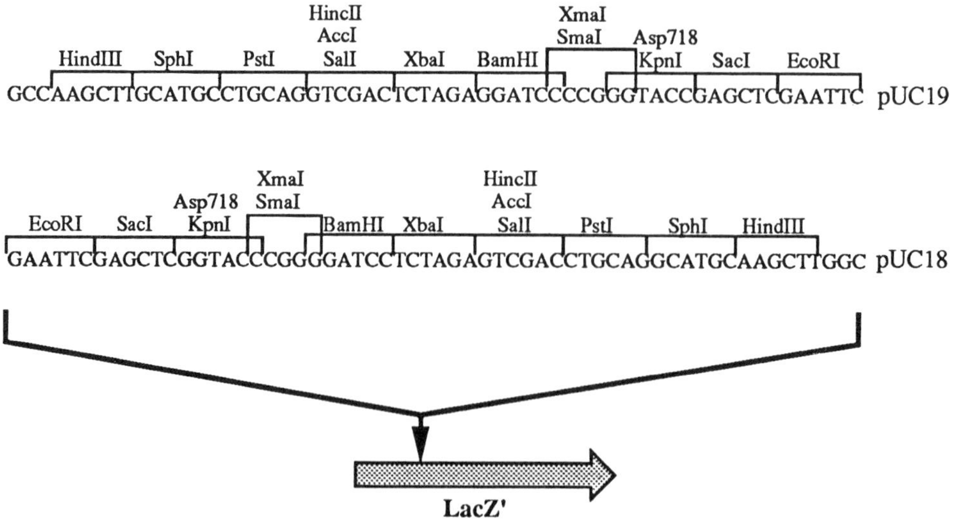

***Figure 2.9* Multiple cloning sites of pUC19 and pUC18.** Note that they contain the same restriction sites but in the opposite orientation. So an *Eco*RI-*Hin*dIII fragment, say, could be cloned into either vector but would have opposite orientations.

each restriction enzyme arranged symmetrically. Subsequent constructs were designed to have unique sites. The latter arrangement means that as well as being able to put restriction fragments with the same site at both ends into the vector as usual, we can cut it with two different enzymes and so enable it to take fragments with a different overhang at each end. (Cleavage of pUC7 with a pair of enzymes will still generate molecules with identical ends.) These vectors come in pairs whose members differ in the orientation of their multiple cloning sites relative to the rest of the vector. So it is possible to determine in advance the orientation of the insert in the vector by appropriate choice of one or the other of the pair. Forcing a particular orientation of vector and insert is known as *forced cloning*. The pUC vectors are therefore a very versatile series. They offer a number of important features:

    a. direct selection for inserts

    b. high copy number

    c. multiple cloning site

    d. forced cloning

    e. controllable promoter

The pUC vectors are probably the most widely used of the "simple" plasmid vectors for *E. coli*.

2. 4 LINKERS, ADAPTORS, AND CASSETTES

2. 4. 1 Linkers

The importance of the pUC vectors owes a great deal to the presence of the multiple cloning site with its ability to accept a wide range of different fragments. A similar feature is offered by molecules called *linkers*. These are short, chemically synthesized molecules that contain a particular restriction enzyme recognition site within the sequence. An example of these, an *Eco*RI linker, is shown in Figure 2.10. Using *Eco*RI linkers, it is possible to clone a blunt-ended insert molecule into a vector carrying an *Eco*RI cloning site. The linkers are themselves blunt-ended molecules and can be joined onto the blunt-ended insert molecule using T4 DNA ligase. Although the reaction – being a blunt-ended ligation – is relatively inefficient, the use of an excess of linker helps to ensure that a large proportion of the insert molecules have linkers on the ends. Some

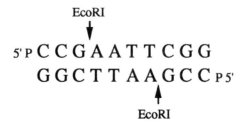

Figure 2.10 An EcoRI linker.

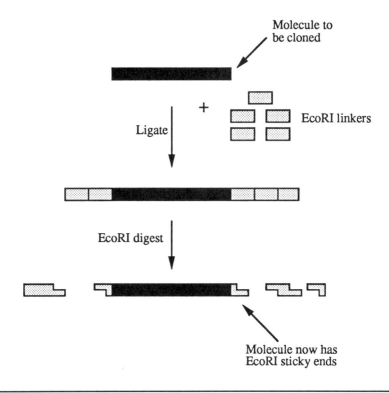

Figure 2.11 Cloning using EcoRI linkers. The linkers are first ligated onto the target molecule in a blunt-ended reaction and are then cleaved with EcoRI.

molecules end up with more than one linker attached to each end, but that is not a problem. The next step is to treat the insert-linker molecules with the appropriate restriction enzyme, which cuts within the linkers to leave a single, cut linker attached to each end of the insert. So the insert now has sticky ends, which can be used for insertion into a restriction site in the usual way. This procedure is summarized in Figure 2.11.

There is a potential problem, though. If the insert itself contains a recognition site for the linker restriction enzyme, the second step of the process in Figure 2.11 will cut the insert as well as the linkers. This is likely to be undesirable. It can be avoided by treatment of the insert, prior to the addition of linkers, with the appropriate methylase – EcoRI methylase, if EcoRI linkers are being used (Section 1.3.4). This renders the molecule insensitive to the restriction enzyme, which will still be able to cut the linker.

Of course, an alternative way of cloning blunt-ended DNA into a vector with EcoRI ends is to avoid using linkers and instead polish up the ends of the cut vector to make them blunt. That could be followed by a blunt-ended ligation of insert DNA into vector. What are the advantages of using linkers? There are three main advantages. One is that it makes better use of the insert and vector DNA, which may be in short supply. Ligation of blunt-ended insert into blunt-ended vector is an inefficient reaction, with much of the insert being wasted. Ligation of blunt-ended linker onto blunt-ended insert can also be inefficient. However, we can use a large excess of linkers (which are in abundant supply, being synthesized on a chemical scale), so that a large proportion of insert acquires linkers and can be efficiently ligated into the vector. The second advantage, which also comes with using an excess of linkers, is that the likelihood of two insert DNA molecules' being ligated to each other (*concatenated*) is reduced. The third advantage comes when it is necessary to cut the insert out of the vector at a later stage. It is unlikely that ligation of a blunt-ended insert into vector that has been cut with *Eco*RI and then polished will regenerate any restriction sites. It is therefore difficult to excise the insert precisely from the vector. However, insert cloned into *Eco*RI-cut vector using *Eco*RI linkers can readily be excised simply by redigestion with *Eco*RI.

There is no reason why a linker should have only one restriction site within it. Linkers that contain a number of sites are available. These are often called polylinkers. The multiple cloning site of the pUC vectors is also often called "the polylinker" and is also available as an oligonucleotide independent of any plasmid.

2. 4. 2 Adaptors

Another development is the group of molecules called adaptors. Examples are given in Figure 2.12. The first shown is an adaptor that is blunt at one end (like a conventional linker) but sticky at the other. It can therefore be ligated, without further digestion, to a blunt-ended molecule to leave a sticky end. Note that in this example the 5' overhanging end is not phosphorylated; this lack of a phosphate group prevents the concatenation of adaptors in the ligation reaction (which would obscure the sticky ends to be used for cloning). Some adaptors (such as the second example in Figure 2.12) are sticky at both ends and can be attached to a molecule that is already sticky-ended, in effect to change the sticky ends. Adaptors may also have extra restriction sites within their sequence.

5'p A G C G G C C G C G
    T C G C C G G C G C T T A A$_{OH}$ 5'

Blunt end/EcoRI sticky-end adaptor

5'p G A T C C G G C A A C G A A G G T A C C A C T G C A
    G C C G T T G C T T C C A T G G T G$_{OH}$ 5'

BamHI sticky-end/PstI sticky-end adaptor

Figure 2.12 **Adaptors.** The upper molecule has a blunt end (left-hand side) and an *Eco*RI sticky end. It can be used to convert a blunt-ended molecule into an *Eco*RI-ended one. The lower molecule has a *Bam*HI end (left-hand side) and a *Pst*I end (right-hand side). It can therefore be ligated onto a molecule with *Bam*HI ends to produce one that has *Pst*I ends.

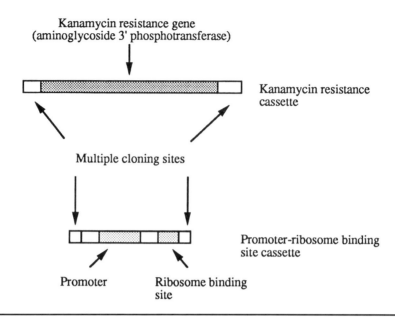

Figure 2.13 Cassettes. The diagram shows examples of an antibiotic resistance cassette (upper) and an expression cassette (lower).

2. 4. 3 Cassettes (cloning cartridges)

Cassettes (cloning cartridges) are a combination of linkers with other sequences. In their simplest form, they consist of an antibiotic resistance gene flanked by DNA that contains multiple cloning sites (Figure 2.13). They can therefore be used as an easy way of incorporating particular selectable markers into DNA molecules. This can be particularly useful as a way of inactivating a cloned gene in the technique of gene disruption (see Section 7.7.1). Some cassettes contain gene expression signals (such as promoters, terminators, etc.) rather than selectable markers. These cassettes are called promoter cassettes (or cartridges), terminator cassettes (or cartridges), and so on.

CHAPTER

3

Other Vector Systems for *E. Coli*

3. 1 INTRODUCTION

So far, we have considered the use of plasmids as cloning vectors for *E. coli*. However, these are not the only molecules able to replicate inside bacterial cells. Bacteriophage viruses must be able to do so as well, and a number of them have been developed for use as cloning vectors. The most widely used are the phages M13 and lambda, but other phages, such as Mu and P1, also have uses. The M13 vectors have a lot in common with the pUC vectors we looked at in Section 2.3.2 and are particularly useful in DNA sequence determination. The lambda vectors are used for more general cloning purposes. There is also a selection of vectors that are hybrids between plasmids and phages. Insertion of viral DNA into a host cell is sometimes called *transfection*, rather than transformation.

3. 2 BACTERIOPHAGE M13 AND ITS USES

3. 2. 1 General biology

Bacteriophage M13 is particularly useful because of its slightly unusual life cycle (summarized in Figure 3.1), which gives us a way of getting single-stranded DNA from double-stranded DNA. It belongs to a group called the

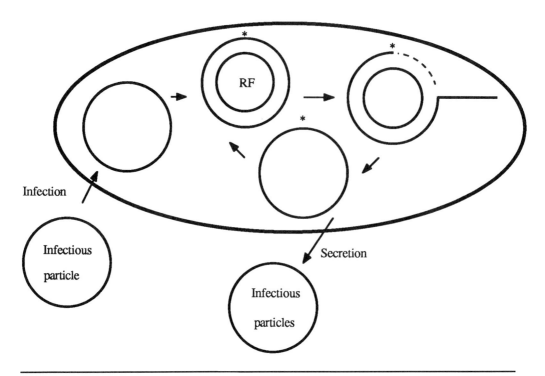

Figure 3.1 Life cycle of bacteriophage M13. RF = replicative form, * indicates the site of nicking or closing by gene II protein, and the dashed region indicates newly synthesized material in rolling circle replication.

filamentous or "skinny" phages, on account of their dimensions. A typical example, fd, is 850 nm x 6 nm. The infectious particle contains single-stranded DNA contained within a protein coat made up primarily of subunits of a single protein species that is the product of gene VIII. There are also a few molecules of the product of gene III. The phage gains entry to the bacterial cells by attaching to the sex pilus before passing its DNA into the cell. It will therefore infect only male cells (i.e., those carrying an F or F' factor, or Hfr strains – in which the F factor has become integrated into the chromosome).

Once inside the cell, the single-stranded molecule (denoted as the + strand) is converted to a double-stranded one called the *replicative form*, or RF. This is done by a means similar to the normal replication process of *E. coli*, using a specific origin of DNA synthesis on the single-stranded molecule for synthesis of the complementary minus strand. The minus strand can then be transcribed to produce viral proteins. The RF DNA can be replicated by a *rolling circle* mode of replication. The product of gene II binds to a specific site on the double-stranded genome and creates a nick in the + strand, generating a free 3'-hydroxyl. This strand is extended by DNA polymerase, displacing the original + strand. After a round of synthesis, the displaced + strand can be separated from the newly synthesized one by another gene II protein nick. This produces a separate + strand, and it is closed by the gene II protein to yield a circular molecule. This can again be converted to RF, which can accumulate to 100 or so copies per cell. As RF accumulates, so does another phage protein, the product of gene V. This blocks not only the synthesis of gene II protein (reducing the synthesis of single strands), but also the conversion of + strands to RF. The single strands are encapsidated in coat proteins and leave the cell. Unlike most phages, virions can be secreted from the cell without causing lysis. A useful feature is that there is no clear constraint on the size of DNA molecule that can be packaged by the coat protein. If DNA molecules longer than normal are to be packaged, more coat protein is attached. This contrasts with phage lambda, for example, which has clear constraints on the amount of phage DNA that can be packaged into each phage particle. Importantly, phage M13 offers us a way of generating *single-stranded* recombinant DNA. Restriction endonucleases will only work on double-stranded molecules, and the plasmids we have encountered so far are double-stranded; the best way of obtaining cloned single-stranded DNA would be to melt the two strands of double-stranded material apart and use them before they reannealed. However, if we can construct double-stranded molecules using M13 RF as a vector and introduce them into *E. coli* by transformation, they will behave there like normal RF DNA and generate single-stranded copies of the same molecules, which can be packaged and released from the cell. So M13 offers a way of converting double-stranded DNA into single-stranded DNA. It is usually much easier and more reliable to use M13 than to prepare single-stranded DNA from double-stranded plasmids by denaturing them.

3. 2. 2 Design of MI3 vectors

The same principles that we saw applied to the design of plasmid vectors (see Section 2.2.1) apply to the design of M13 vectors. We need an origin of replication. The phage has its own, so that presents no difficulty. There is also no problem over a selectable marker as the phage is, in a sense, a selectable marker itself. Cells that take up phage DNA will produce more phage and become a focus for infection of other cells. Plating out the cells from a transformation will therefore generate a *lawn* (a uniform layer of cells) peppered with holes (*plaques*) arising from cells that have taken up phage DNA molecules and produced more phage, which have infected surrounding cells. Although M13 does not actually lyse the cells it infects, it retards their growth, so the plaques that are seen are not true phage plaques (which arise from cell lysis), but areas of slow growth. The cell division time of infected *E. coli* increases from 20 minutes under optimum conditions to more than 2 hours upon M13 infection. Because the plaques result from slow growth rather than genuine lysis, they are sometimes known as *pseudoplaques*.

The ability of phage to infect cells, produce more phage, and consequently produce a plaque, depends on inserting DNA without affecting any of the phage genes necessary for replication. The M13 genome is quite tightly packed (Figure 3.2), and there are therefore rather few places available to insert DNA. One available site is in an intergenic spacer between genes II and IV. The *lacZ* minigene and multiple cloning region (discussed in Section 2.3.2) have been incorporated here. This modification brings with it all the advantages of the multiple cloning site – such as the ability to accept a wide range of restriction fragments and to force cloning in a particular orientation – as well as the added

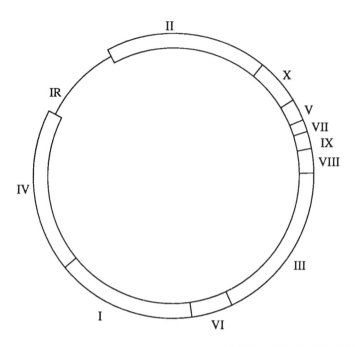

Figure 3.2 **Bacteriophage M13 genome. I–X** indicate the genes, **IR** indicates the intergenic region where DNA can be inserted.

advantage of direct colour selection for the presence of an insert afforded by the *lacZ* cloning system. For the *lacZ* system to work, the F' plasmid carrying the rest of the beta-galactosidase gene must be present in the host. (An F' is also needed to ensure that the host produces the sex pilus required for M13 phage infection.) After transformation, the host cells are mixed with soft agar, X-Gal, and IPTG before plating out and incubation to form a lawn. Cells that have taken up phage DNA will give rise to plaques, and if the *lacZ'* coding sequence within the phage is intact, the plaques will have a blue colour distinguishable from the off-white background. Figure 3.3 shows the organization of some of the M13 phages used for cloning. Just as with the pUC plasmids, there is a series of phages, in this case designated "mp." The cloning region in M13mp18 is identical to that in pUC18, and so on. The requirements for M13 hosts are similar to those for pUC plasmids (indeed the same strains are generally used), which were discussed in Section 2.3.2. Other regions for the incorporation of DNA (for example, between genes VIII and III) have also been exploited, but these vectors are less widely used.

Other requirements for vectors (discussed in Section 2.2.1) are also satisfied by M13 – at 7.3 kb, the vector is small enough to be handled easily, and the RF has a high copy number inside the cell. With M13, the intracellular copy number is less important than with plasmid vectors, as we are usually interested in the single-stranded DNA in the phage secreted from infected cells. Whereas intracellular plasmid DNA is collected by cell lysis, as described in Section 1.5 (and this is the approach taken for preparing RF DNA for cloning purposes), the single-stranded DNA must be collected rather differently. An infected culture is set up, and after a while the cells are removed by centrifugation, leaving the phage in the super-

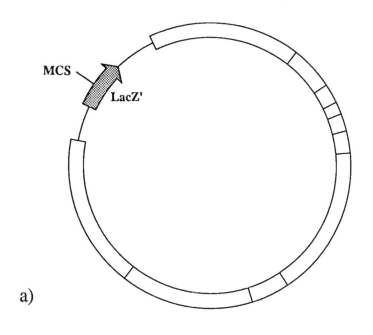

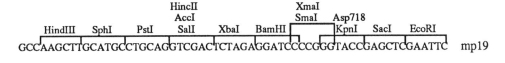

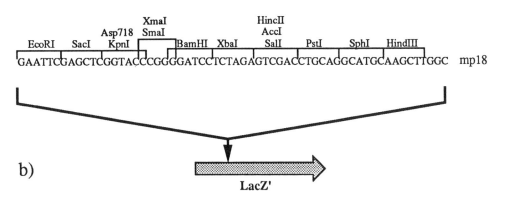

Figure 3.3 **M13 vectors.** Panel (**a**) shows the position of the *lacZ'* minigene and multiple cloning site (MCS). Panel (**b**) shows the position of restriction sites within the multiple cloning sites of phages M13mp19 and M13mp18.

natant. The phage are then precipitated, usually by the addition of polyethylene glycol and sodium chloride (although other methods are possible, too) followed by centrifugation. The phage pellet is resuspended, and the protein is removed with phenol to leave single-stranded DNA in solution. This is then recovered by precipitation. Under standard conditions, several micrograms of single-stranded DNA can be obtained from a few millilitres of a culture of infected cells.

3. 2. 3 DNA Sequencing and M13

1. DNA Sequencing. By far the most important application of M13 cloning is in DNA sequence determination by the *Sanger* method – also called the *dideoxy* or *chain-termination* method. This relies on the use of chain-terminating inhibitors of DNA synthesis, the 2',3'-dideoxynucleoside triphosphates (ddNTPs). These are shown in Figure 3.4, together with the 2'-deoxynucleoside triphosphates (dNTPs), which are the normal components for DNA synthesis. A growing DNA chain is extended in the 5'–3' direction by nucleophilic attack of the 3'-hydroxyl group on the alpha-phosphate of the next dNTP. The ddNTP analogues can be incorporated into a growing DNA chain in the usual way, but since they lack the 3'-hydroxyl group (it is replaced by a hydrogen), they will not allow any further synthesis. They are therefore chain-terminating inhibitors.

The method is summarized in Figure 3.5:

a. Obtain the DNA to be sequenced in single-stranded form.

b. Anneal to it a short complementary oligonucleotide. This is the *primer* for subsequent DNA synthesis.

c. Divide the mix into four aliquots, and add to each: DNA polymerase (Section 1.3.2), all four dNTPs (one of which – the same one in each tube – is radioactively labelled), and one of the four ddNTPs (a different one to each tube).

d. Incubate for a suitable period. (In some protocols there is a short preincubation before the addition of ddNTPs.) During the incubation, DNA syn-

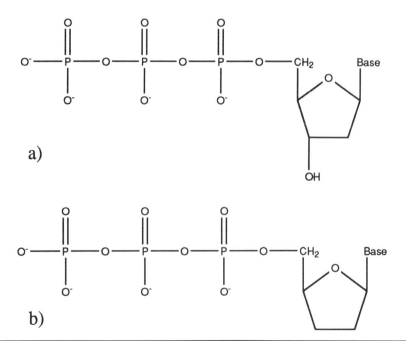

Figure 3.4 **2'-deoxynucleoside triphosphate (a) and 2',3'-dideoxynucleoside triphosphate (b).**

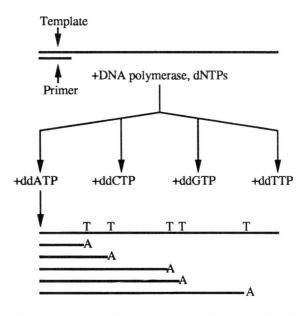

Figure 3.5 **The principle of DNA sequencing.** The figure shows the products of synthesis from template and primer in the presence of ddATP, resulting in termination opposite T residues in the template.

thesis will take place in each tube. In the tube to which 2',3'-dideoxyadenosine triphosphate (ddATP) was added, synthesis will be terminated opposite T residues because of the incorporation of the dideoxynucleotide. Because some dATP was also present, only a fraction of the molecules being synthesized will terminate at any given A (or opposite any given T). The actual fraction will depend on the ratio of ddATP to dATP in the reaction mix. So this tube now contains a series of radioactively labelled DNA molecules, all with the same 5' end – the primer – but with different 3' ends (all ending with A). Similarly, the tube to which ddCTP was added contains a nested set of molecules all ending in C's (opposite G's), and so on.

e. The contents of each reaction are electrophoresed in a denaturing polyacrylamide gel, in adjacent lanes, and the positions of the radioactive DNA molecules are determined autoradiographically. A schematic example is shown in Figure 3.6. The bands in the gel correspond to DNA molecules that have terminated at a particular position. In the example given, the smallest molecules (i.e., those that have moved furthest in the gel) end in C, the next smallest in A, and so on. So the sequence would read (5'–3') CA (or TG on the opposite strand). These gels can be read "manually", although automated and semiautomated systems are also available. Because of the amount and type of information generated, the sequences are generally stored and manipulated by computer.

The DNA does not have to be radioactively labelled. Fluorescent labels are an attractive alternative. One system uses four different primers that have the

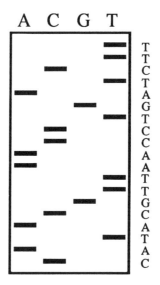

Figure 3.6 Schematic representation of a DNA sequencing gel. The gel is read from the bottom, and the interpretation is given alongside.

same sequence but different fluorescent labels – a different one for each reaction. The reaction products are then mixed and run in the *same* lane in the gel. A fluorescence detector records the molecules as they pass a particular point in the gel and determines whether they are from the A, G, C, or T reactions according to the fluorescence tag. The information is then fed directly into a computer. This procedure allows data collection in real time, without the need to stop the electrophoresis, to process the gel for autoradiography, and so forth. It can therefore save a considerable amount of time. Not only can the detection system be automated, but it is possible to automate the sequencing reactions by using robot pipettors. There are other modifications to the technique, such as using fluorescent labelled nucleotides or having separate labelling and termination stages. One of the chief technical difficulties encountered is the formation of secondary structure in the template or the newly synthesized strand. It may be possible to avoid formation of secondary structure by using different polymerases (Section 1.3.2) or different nucleotides (e.g., 2'-deoxy-7-deaza-GTP).

2. Application of M13. The main requirements for template DNA generated for sequencing are therefore

   a. that it should be single-stranded, and

   b. that before the beginning of the region to be sequenced, there should be some "known" sequence for which a primer can be made.

These requirements can readily be met using M13 since

   a. single-stranded DNA can easily be purified from phage particles, and

   b. the sequence adjacent to the multiple cloning site is independent of what is inserted at the site, so the same *universal primer* can always be used.

3. Cloning strategies. A single set of DNA sequencing reactions run on a gel will give a limited amount of DNA sequence information. The amount is determined by the number of nucleotides that can be resolved on a single gel, as well as by the sequencing reactions. With a standard gel system, it may be possible to resolve 300 bp or so, although the use of field strength gradient gels (Section 1.6.4) will generate more information. The sequence of a piece of target DNA must therefore be built up in short runs of up to 300 bp or so. Ideally, these runs should cover both strands and overlap each other. There are four main ways of building up this information. They are summarized in Figure 3.7, and descriptions of the four methods follow:

a. CLONING OF RESTRICTION FRAGMENTS. Sequence information can be built up by the cloning of restriction fragments. Restriction enzymes are used to cut the target DNA fragment into smaller subfragments, which are inserted into the M13 multiple cloning site and sequenced. Each subfragment will not necessarily be sequenced in its entirety but will be sequenced just as far as the resolution of the gels permits. If the location of each sequenced subfragment is known, it is easier to piece together the

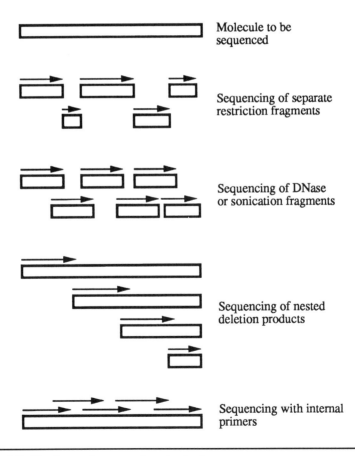

Figure 3.7 Cloning and sequencing strategies.

information gathered in each sequencing run. However, prior information about the target molecule (i.e., the restriction map) may not be available. One can still use restriction enzymes in the absence of a map to generate subfragments whose locations are not known at the outset. (These are sometimes called "random" fragments, but that is a misnomer, since they are still produced by specific digestion.) Enzymes with 4-nucleotide recognition sites are the most suitable, since the expected average size of the fragments they generate is close to the expected amount of sequence yielded from each run, thus maximizing the amount of information obtained from any one cloning.

So the target DNA is cut with the enzyme, and the fragments are shotgun cloned into M13 and sequenced. In order to generate overlaps between the stretches of sequence obtained, it is necessary to do at least two sets of sequencing experiments, each with a different restriction enzyme. The sequences obtained are analysed by computer to find overlapping regions, which allows the pieces to be assembled. The main disadvantage with this approach lies in the unequal sizes of the fragments generated – they will not all be the expected average of 256 base pairs. Some will be much smaller, and some larger. The small fragments are likely to be cloned preferentially, and each sequencing run gives little information. Because of the preferential cloning, a large number of independent clones may prove to have identical small inserts. Finding clones with large inserts may require sequencing a lot of clones, and in any case, it is not possible to sequence the large clones in their entirety. Using the strategy of sequencing restriction fragments, it is therefore difficult to sequence any parts of the target DNA that are particularly underendowed with restriction sites.

In practice, directed cloning and random cloning are often employed together. In the early stages of a project, random fragments may be used to generate a partial sequence of the target DNA. This information is then used to identify particular restriction fragments that can be used to obtain more sequence information to "fill in the gaps".

b. CLONING OF SONICATION OR DNASE FRAGMENTS. We saw in Section 1.2 how sonication or treatment with nonspecific endonucleases can be used to generate fragments of a DNA molecule regardless of the distribution of restriction sites. Both techniques are suited to the generation of fragments for sequencing, with sonication being the approach preferred by many. The extent of sonication is adjusted appropriately and is combined with electrophoretic fractionation and recovery from the gel to obtain fragments that are slightly too large to be sequenced completely (for a reason that will be explained shortly). Although some of the fragments may have blunt ends, others will not, and there is no way of predicting what ends the fragments will have. The ends of the fragments are therefore polished (Sections 1.3.2 and 1.3.3) before the fragments are cloned into a site in the M13 vector able to receive blunt ends (e.g., the *Sma*I or *Hinc*II sites). The inserts are sequenced, and the overall sequence is built up by computer analysis.

Two precautions are necessary in the cloning and sequencing strategy just discussed. One is necessitated by the possibility that two sonication subfragments may be ligated in tandem into the M13 cloning site. Ligation of the subfragments does not regenerate any identifiable restriction site, so there is no way of detecting that the ligation has occurred. If the sequencing run proceeds entirely through one subfragment and into the next, two stretches of sequence will be recorded as contiguous when they are not. However, if all the individual subfragments cloned are slightly too long to be fully sequenced, then none of the sequencing runs will be able to cross this boundary. Ligation of noncontiguous fragments is not a problem when using restriction subfragments, as described earlier in Section 3.2.3 (see "Cloning of restriction fragments"), since such a ligation can usually be detected by the regeneration within the sequence of the restriction site for the enzyme used for cloning.

As well as adjusting subfragment sizes as just described, it is necessary to avoid overrepresentation in the subfragments of the sequences from the ends of the initial fragment. If a linear molecule is used for the sonication, then the sequences at each end will always be adjacent to an end after fragmentation (because they were adjacent to an end before fragmentation!) and will therefore have a disproportionately high chance of being cloned and sequenced. This problem can be avoided by circularization of the linear molecule before sonication, although noncontiguous sequences will again be placed together. This time – as a result of the circularization – the restriction site utilized to generate the linear molecule will regenerate, and the presence of noncontiguous sequences can therefore be detected quite easily by screening the sequences determined for that site.

c. NESTED DELETIONS. Rather than fragment the target molecule and clone the bits, it may be more convenient to generate a set of nested deletions of the molecule by exonuclease activity. Such a set of deletions brings regions from further and further inside the target fragment within the reach of the primer annealing site. One approach is first to clone the entire fragment into M13 and then prepare RF of the recombinant molecule. RF is then linearized and degraded sequentially, as described in Section 1.3.3.

d. INTERNAL PRIMERS. The fourth approach does not require fragmentation of the target molecule. The entire molecule is cloned into the multiple cloning site, and single-stranded DNA is prepared. The first sequencing run gives information on the sequence close to the end of the target molecule. Using this information, an oligonucleotide is synthesized that will anneal within the insert. This oligonucleotide is used as a sequencing primer instead of the universal primer to sequence further into the insert. On the basis of the sequence generated, another primer can be synthesized, and so on. Drawbacks to this method are the cost of synthesizing the primers, the delay between each step as primers are synthesized, and the need to clone large fragments into M13, which may lead to the occurrence and propagation of deletion mutants. The approach is often used to finish off a project that has been almost completed using strategies (a), (b), or (c).

4. Other applications of M13 cloning. M13 is of use whenever there is a requirement for single-stranded DNA. As well as DNA sequencing, this includes site-directed mutagenesis, which will be discussed later (Section 7.5.1). M13 is also of particular use in generating probes for RNA analysis. Probes can be prepared that are specific for RNA transcripts from either strand of DNA. These applications are outside the scope of this book, but more information can be obtained from specialized laboratory manuals. M13 is also used in *phage display* systems, described in Section 3.2.4.

5. Double-stranded DNA sequencing. Although single-stranded DNA usually gives the best results in sequencing procedures, double-stranded DNA can also be used. The strands are first separated by heat treatment or by raising the pH. The denatured DNA is then allowed to anneal to the primer. However, the complementary DNA strands may also reanneal to each other rather than to the primer; this reannealing will regenerate the double-stranded molecule, which is unsuitable for sequencing. It is therefore important to adjust the conditions (primer-template ratio, annealing conditions, time allowed for annealing, etc.) to optimize the primer's annealing. The pUC plasmids are often used for sequencing with double-stranded DNA, because the same primers can be used as for M13.

Double-stranded DNA can also be used in the chemical sequencing method developed by Maxam and Gilbert. Linear DNA fragments (e.g., restriction fragments), labelled at one end on one strand, are treated in a number of different reactions with chemicals that result in cleavage at particular nucleotides. This generates sets of radiolabelled molecules with the products of a given reaction all terminating at known nucleotides. The sequence can therefore be deduced by electrophoresis and autoradiography in a method similar to the one employed in Sanger sequencing. More details can be found in general biochemical textbooks or in specialized sequencing manuals.

3.2.4 M13 Derivatives

1. Phage-plasmid hybrids. The requirements for a molecule to be replicated as single-stranded DNA and packaged into a phage coat are modest. All that is necessary is for the molecule to contain the viral origin of DNA synthesis, as long as the other functions can be provided by other phage DNA molecules within the cell, acting in *trans*. This fact allowed the construction of M13-plasmid hybrid vectors, sometimes called *phagemid* (and also sometimes called *phasmid* or *plage*, although the term phasmid is often used for lambda phage derivatives, described in Section 3.3.4). Plasmids that carry the M13 replication origin in addition to a regular origin of double-stranded DNA synthesis can be replicated either as double-stranded DNA from the latter or, if the appropriate proteins (such as gene II protein) are provided from a *helper phage* also replicating within the cell, as single-stranded DNA. The single-stranded DNA produced is then packaged. Examples of these vectors are the plasmids pUC118, 119, and 120. They will be replicated as plasmids until the cell containing them is co-infected with a helper phage such as M13KO7, which provides the proteins for single-stranded DNA synthesis and packaging. M13KO7 is an M13 phage that has been modified, most importantly by the incorporation of a plasmid replication origin. Replication from this origin allows the helper phage to be present in a high copy number per cell and therefore to provide larger quantities of the

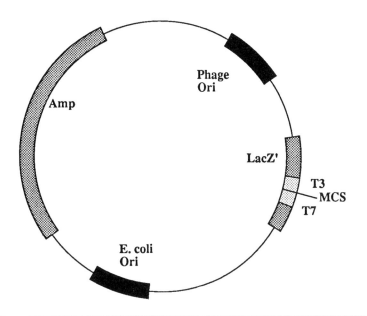

Figure 3.8 pBluescriptIIKS⁺ (3.0 kb). The phagemid contains an ampicillin resistance selectable marker (Amp) and origins (Ori) for double-stranded replication (E. coli) and for single-stranded DNA synthesis (Phage), the latter for use when cells containing the vector are co-infected with a suitable helper phage. There are a multiple cloning site (MCS) in the LacZ' minigene (allowing blue/white selection for the presence of an insert), and phage T3 and T7 promoters for transcription of inserted DNA sequences.

proteins that are required to replicate and package the phagemid molecule. M13KO7 also contains a kanamycin resistance gene to allow for selection for the presence of the phage. (Of course it is possible that the M13KO7 helper phage may be packaged too, but in practice, packaged phagemid molecules are found to be in a 100-fold excess over the helper phage.) Another example of these vectors is the pBluescript series, which includes pBluescriptIIKS⁺, shown in Figure 3.8. This series of plasmids contains, in addition, promoters from the *E. coli* bacteriophages T3 or T7, which are useful for expressing cloned sequences (see Section 8.2.2). The main advantage of the phagemid system is that it can be used to provide single- or double-stranded material without any recloning.

2. Phage display vectors. An important use of filamentous phage is in *phage display* systems. Here, coding sequences are inserted into one of the coat protein genes, often gene III. The result is that the phage are generated with a hybrid form of this protein, which is a fusion of the normal protein sequence and the protein product of the inserted sequence (assuming the inserted sequence has the same reading frame as gene III). The phage are secreted from the cell, with this extra material "displayed" on the outside. Fusions with gene VIII can also be engineered, resulting in the display of many more copies of the extra peptide than are obtained with gene III, as the former is present in more copies per phage particle. These display vectors have many uses, such as the screening of libraries by *panning,* as described in Section 5.2.1, and for vaccine production.

3. 3   BACTERIOPHAGE LAMBDA

3. 3. 1   General Biology

In order to understand the cloning vectors based on bacteriophage lambda, some general knowledge of lambda biology is necessary. A simplified map of the lambda genome is shown in Figure 3.9. Lambda is an example of a *temperate* phage. After infecting a host cell, temperate phage can either replicate and cause lysis (the *lytic* pathway) or integrate their genome into the host cell's to generate a lysogen (the *lysogenic* pathway). At a later stage the lysogen may be activated, or *induced*. The phage genome is then expressed, the phage is excised from the host genome, more phage are produced, and the host is lysed. Which pathway is followed, and under what circumstances a lysogen is induced, depend on the physiological state of the host cell.

Upon infection, two promoters become active (Figure 3.9). These are P_R and P_L, for *rightward* and *leftward* transcription respectively. They give rise to the *immediate early* transcripts, which terminate at rightward and leftward terminators, t_R and t_L. These transcripts direct synthesis of the *N* and *cro* gene products. The N protein allows the t_R and t_L terminators to be overridden, so subsequent transcription extends through into the surrounding regions, including *cII* and *cIII*. The extended transcripts are termed the *delayed early* transcripts and include those for the proteins of DNA replication. The *cII* and *cIII* gene products, but particularly *cII*, activate another promoter, P_{RE} (promoter for repressor establishment), and it is now that the choice is made between following the lytic or the lysogenic mode.

1.   The lysogenic mode. The key factor in the decision between lysis and lysogeny is the stability of the *cII* gene product, which is protected by the CIII protein against degradation by host proteases. (Levels of host proteases in turn depend upon a range of parameters, including cAMP levels.) If the *cII* gene product is stable, then CII-stimulated transcription from P_{RE} leads to the production of the CI protein. This is a repressor molecule that inactivates P_R and

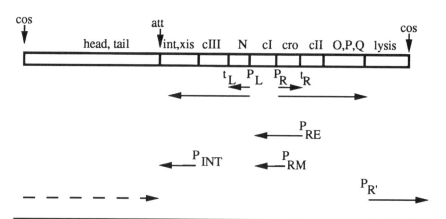

Figure 3.9 Simplified map of the bacteriophage lambda genome, with the promoters and transcripts arising from them.

P_L and therefore switches off the expression of the rest of the lambda genome. The CII protein and its transcript also interfere with the synthesis of Cro and Q – both of which are needed for lytic growth – and thus add a further block to the lytic pathway. The CII protein *also* activates transcription from another promoter (called P_{INT}), which leads to production of the Int protein. This protein, in conjunction with host proteins, mediates a site-specific recombination event across a site in the phage (called *att*) and a homologous sequence in the bacterial chromosome, integrating the phage. However, CI repressor protein soon switches off the expression of *cII* and *cIII*, so *int* expression ceases too. The phage is thus integrated by a brief pulse of *int* expression, and phage genes are switched off by CI. The integrated lambda genome would now be completely silent transcriptionally were it not for another promoter, P_{RM} (promoter for repressor maintenance), which is activated by low levels of the CI protein (and inhibited by high levels) and leads to synthesis of further CI protein, ensuring that the repressed state of the rest of the phage genome is maintained. The integrated phage is called a *prophage*, and the bacterial cell containing it is a *lysogen*. Lysogens are immune to further infection by the same phage, because the incoming genome is immediately repressed by the levels of CI protein already present in the host cell cytoplasm. Plaques of lambda on an *E. coli* lawn will therefore usually be *turbid* because of the growth of a few lysogens in the presence of the lambda phage in the plaque. Mutant phage that are unable to form lysogens (for example, as a result of inactivation of the *cI, cII,* or *cIII* genes) will therefore form clear plaques. (In fact, the "*c*" in those genes stands for *clear plaques*.)

2. **The lytic cycle**. If the CII protein is not stable under the conditions prevailing at the time of infection, P_{RE} is not activated, little repressor can be synthesized, and transcription of the rest of the phage genome can continue. The Cro protein that is produced reinforces this switch by inactivating the P_{RM} promoter, ensuring that no CI repressor is produced. The Q protein that is the product of delayed early gene expression then acts to allow expression from $P_{R'}$ (by a method analogous to that used by N), and the late genes are expressed, to produce coat (head and tail) proteins, allowing assembly of functional phage and cell lysis.

3. **Induction of a lysogen**. Induction of a lysogen will take place if the level of the CI in the cell falls, perhaps by specific breakdown by the host RecA protease as a response to DNA damage. The fall in the level of CI lifts the repression of P_R and P_L, allowing expression of phage genes. These include *int* and *xis,* which together lead to phage excision. Replication and coat protein synthesis take place, as with the lytic cycle; phage particles are then assembled and the host is lysed.

4. **Replication and packaging of DNA.** Lambda DNA replication usually takes place in two phases. In the first phase, replication is in the bidirectional *theta* mode to generate additional circular DNA molecules. In the second phase, replication transfers to a *rolling circle* mode with a single replication fork and yields concatemeric molecules (Figure 3.10). These are needed for assembly into mature phage particles. Assembly is dependent upon the presence on the concatenated molecule of sites called *cos* (refer to Figure 3.9), flanking the region to

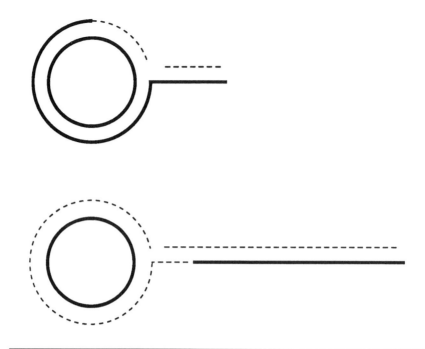

Figure 3.10 Rolling circle replication. DNA synthesis (dashed line) displaces a single strand that can also serve as a template for synthesis. As synthesis progresses (lower panel), concatenated complete double-stranded genomes are spooled off.

be packaged. One genome's length of phage DNA is inserted into the phage head, and this brings adjacent *cos* sites together. Staggered cleavage of the DNA then takes place at the *cos* sites and generates 12-base overhanging ends. Without the *cos* site, packaging would not be possible. The size of the phage head imposes constraints on the amount of DNA that can be packaged into each phage particle, setting both a maximum and a minimum limit. The wild-type lambda genome is 48.5 kb, and molecules between approximately 40 kb and 52 kb can be efficiently packaged (provided they have a *cos* site, of course).

3. 3. 2 Cloning in lambda

1. Insertion vectors. These are the simplest vectors. DNA is inserted into a single restriction site, which must be in a nonessential gene to maintain phage viability. Because of the upper limit on the size of DNA that can be packaged in the lambda head, there is a corresponding limit of a few kilobases on the amount of extra DNA that can be included. Lambda gt10 and gt11 are examples of insertion vectors and illustrate the limited amount of DNA they can accept (see Figure 3.11). Lambda gt10 has a unique *Eco*RI site, within the *cI* repressor gene, and can accept inserts up to 7.6 kb in size. This is a bit larger than inserts that wild-type phage would be able to accept, because there is a small deletion elsewhere in the genome of gt10. The presence of the inserts can be detected by the consequent inactivation of *cI* (see "Selection of recombinants" later in Section 3.2.2). Lambda gt11 contains a *lacZ* gene with a unique *Eco*RI site. Protein-coding DNA sequences inserted into this can be expressed as a fusion with the LacZ protein (see Section 8.3.4). (The *cI/cro* control region of gt11 has in fact been replaced by that from another phage, 434, but the organization and function of the gt11 genome both remain the same.)

2. Substitution or replacement vectors. In these vectors, a portion of the phage genome is removed by restriction digestion and is replaced with the DNA to be cloned. Much of the central region of lambda is not necessary for lytic growth and can be removed. The region includes the repressor gene, so the lysogenic mode of growth is no longer possible. The regions left include those responsible for phage DNA replication, the phage coat and its assembly, and cell lysis. About 20 kb of the phage genome can therefore be removed and be replaced with a piece of inserted DNA, which is called the *stuffer* fragment. The stuffer fragment is often generated by partial digestion with an enzyme with a 4- base-pair recognition site (see Section 1.2.1). Figure 3.11 shows a typical substitution vector, EMBL4. It contains two copies of a multiple cloning site, flanking the region to be removed. Digestion with an enzyme cutting within the multiple cloning site will separate the central region from the left and right flanking sections (or *arms*).

Before we can ligate in the stuffer fragment, it is necessary to take steps to stop the central portion from being religated to the arms again. This can be done by cleavage of the central portion with a second enzyme or by physical separation. If a second enzyme is used, it must cut within the central region, but not within the arms, so *Sal*I could be used for EMBL4 previously cut with *Bam*HI. It may not be necessary to remove the fragments generated, because the multimolecular reaction needed to regenerate the original phage will be so infrequent. Alternatively, if the second cuts are at sites very close to the first, such as

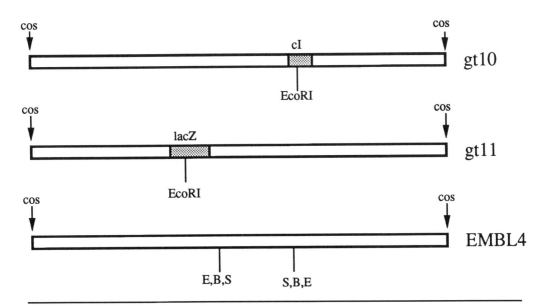

Figure 3.11 Examples of lambda phage vectors. In gt10 and gt11, there are *Eco*RI sites in the *cl* and *lacZ* genes respectively (shaded) for insertion of DNA. EMBL4 is a substitution or replacement vector, from which a substantial nonessential region of the molecule can be removed by digestion with *Eco*RI (E), *Bam*HI (B), or *Sal*I (S).

with a *Bam*HI digest of EMBL4 followed by a *Sal*I digest, the small fragments generated may be too small to be precipitated by ethanol. Precipitation of the DNA after the second cut and recovery of the pellet would therefore yield the arms (with *Bam*HI ends), along with a part of the central region (with *Sal*I ends) that could no longer be ligated into them.

Physical separation can be done either in an agarose gel or by centrifugation in a sucrose density gradient (which separates DNA molecules by size, in contrast to CsCl gradients). The arms are then recovered from the gel or the gradient. Generally, the DNA recovered from the gel is less efficient in ligation reactions than that recovered from sucrose gradients, so the latter technique is preferred.

3. Packaging *in vitro*. It is possible to introduce recombinant lambda molecules into a host by transformation with naked DNA, as we do with plasmids. However, this process is very inefficient, and we can improve it by orders of magnitude if we package the DNA *in vitro* into phage coats and use the phage's normal DNA infection process to get the DNA into the host cell. Packaging *in vitro* is essentially just a matter of incubating lambda DNA in a concatemeric configuration with a lysate of lambda-infected cells. This lysate would contain the lambda proteins (and host proteins such as chaperones) needed for phage assembly and should therefore be able to package the added recombinant DNA, too. However, in practice it is not that simple, as there would be a high background of nonrecombinant lambda phage produced from the packaging extract (which would contain lambda DNA, as well as the packaging proteins). The usual approach is to use two separate strains, carrying lambda prophage with chain termination mutations in different genes for coat components (the *D* and *E* genes). It is convenient if the prophage have a temperature-sensitive CI repressor, so they can be induced by heat shock. On induction, packaging proteins are produced in each strain; however, no packaging can occur because neither strain is producing the full complement of proteins needed. Lysates of the cells from both strains are then prepared and mixed. The mixed lysate has all the proteins needed for packaging, which can now start. At this point, the DNA we want to package is therefore added.

It is important to use suitable strains for packaging. They should carry prophage with the following features:

a. AMBER CHAIN TERMINATION MUTATIONS IN THE *D* AND *E* GENES, which encode components of the head.

b. THE *cI*857 TEMPERATURE-SENSITIVE REPRESSOR PROTEIN GENE, which allows control of prophage induction by heating.

c. AMBER CHAIN TERMINATION MUTATIONS IN THE *S* GENE. These mutations block cell lysis and allow the growth of cells containing very high levels of packaging proteins. We can then lyse the cells artificially.

d. *red* MUTATION. This mutation blocks a phage-encoded recombination pathway and therefore decreases the likelihood that recombination (and rearrangement) of DNA will take place *in vitro* during packaging. The lysogenic strains also usually carry the *recA* mutation, which largely blocks the *E. coli* recombination pathway and further reduces the likelihood of rearrangement *in vitro*.

e. A DELETION IN THE *b* REGION. This prevents excision of the prophage on induction and therefore reduces the amount of endogenous phage DNA in the packaging mix and the consequent level of background nonrecombinant phage after packaging.

Because packaging phage molecules requires the presence of *cos* sites on each side of the region to be packaged, the optimal substrate for packaging is a (left arm–insert–right arm)$_n$ concatemer, and the molar ratio of arms to insert should therefore be adjusted appropriately for the ligation. This is usually done empirically by carrying out small-scale ligation and packaging reactions. When the optimum ratio is established, a large-scale reaction is carried out. Note that the left and right arms are held together in the concatemer by annealing at the *cos* site. Once packaged, the phage DNA is introduced into *E. coli* by infection, as with lambda phage generated by more conventional means. The whole process is summarized in Figure 3.12.

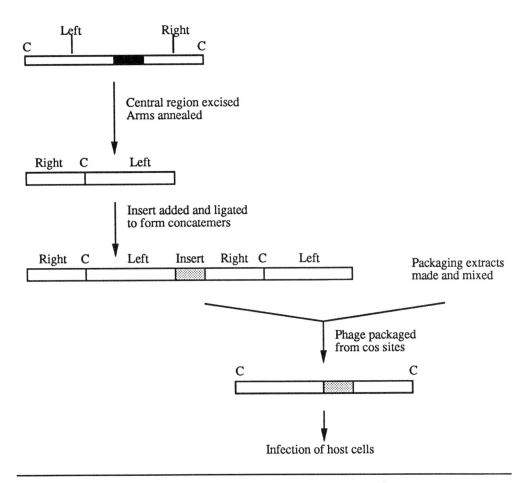

Figure 3.12 **Summary of cloning into a lambda substitution vector.** C = *cos* site.

4. Selection of recombinants. As with M13 cloning, uptake of a phage DNA molecule is marked by the formation of a plaque on an *E. coli* lawn. It is necessary to be able to distinguish between phages carrying an insert and those lacking one. There are many ways of going about this, depending on the particular phage used. They include

a. SELECTION FOR *cI* FUNCTION. The CI repressor protein is required for the formation of lysogens. Phage in which the *cI* gene has been inactivated are therefore unable to form lysogens and will produce clear plaques rather than turbid ones. (Plaque turbidity is caused by the presence in the plaque of lysogenic cells that are immune from further infection because of the CI protein in their cytoplasm.) So if the cloning site (in an insertion vector) or the removed region (in a replacement vector) involves the *cI* gene, recombinant phage will be *cI*⁻ and can be recognized by their forming clear plaques, whereas nonrecombinant ones will be *cI*⁺ and form turbid plaques. This selection can be enhanced using an *hflA* (high frequency of lysogenization) mutant host, in which CII stability is enhanced. This causes lysogenization to take place so efficiently that phage capable of forming lysogens do so in preference to entering the lytic pathway and fail to form plaques at all. Only phage that are incapable of forming lysogens (i.e., those that have lost *cI* function) will form plaques.

b. *lac* SELECTION. Some insertional vectors have a cloning site in a *lacZ* gene that has been introduced into the phage genome. Insertion of DNA into the cloning site therefore inactivates the production of beta-galactosidase in infected cells, and plaques on a lawn on medium containing X-Gal and IPTG will be colourless. Plaques from phage lacking an insert will be blue. A similar approach can be used with replacement vectors, if the region replaced carries the appropriate part of a *lacZ* gene. Phage with an insert will give colourless plaques; those without will give blue ones. The *lacZ* can be either a minigene (as with the pUC vectors described in Section 2.3.2) or an intact gene.

c. *spi* SELECTION. The use of *spi* selection relies on a slightly esoteric piece of phage biology. The *red* and *gam* gene products of phage lambda (an exonuclease involved in recombination and a protein inactivating the *E. coli* recBCD nuclease respectively) inhibit its growth in *E. coli* cells that are lysogenic for the bacteriophage P2. However, *red*⁻*gam*⁻ phage can grow in a P2 lysogen. Because the *red* and *gam* genes are removed during cloning in replacement phages, phage that have acquired an insert will be able to grow on a lawn of P2-lysogenic *E. coli*, and those that haven't won't. Recombinant phage can therefore be selected by plating on a P2 lysogen. (For propagation of the phage for subsequent DNA preparation, a host lacking the P2 prophage is used, as growth is much better.) Phage that are *red*⁻*gam*⁻ are often designated *spi*⁻, and others denoted *spi*⁺ (**s**ensitive to **P2 i**nhibition).

Unfortunately, *red*⁻*gam*⁻ phage produce rather few virions in infected cells. This is because the *recBCD* nuclease (which is inhibited by the Gam protein) blocks rolling circle replication. *Gam*⁻ phage are therefore unable to inhibit the action of RecBCD, and are therefore unable to carry out rolling circle replication. Therefore, the only way concatemers (which are needed for the production of packaged phage) can be formed is by recombination between the circular molecules formed by *theta* replication. Recombination between two circular molecules would generate a circular dimer for packaging. However, the host recombination enzymes may not work on lambda DNA (if it does not contain the necessary recombination initiation sites, called *chi* sites), and the phage recombination system (which relies on the *red* gene) is missing. The only way a useful level of recombination (and concatemer formation) can be ensured is to include the *red* gene or a *chi* site in the phage. Many phage, such as EMBL4, have *chi* sites. The insert DNA may by chance also have them, but it is unwise to rely on this; phages with inserts that lack a *chi* site will be at a selective disadvantage.

5. **Amplification.** Amplification is often useful when constructing libraries in lambda, especially if the number of phage produced after packaging *in vitro* is low. The procedure, which should not be confused with chloramphenicol amplification of plasmids (Section 2.2.1), is simply the propagation of the phage in *E. coli*. Each phage that infects an *E. coli* cell will give rise to many more phage after the cell is lysed, so the result is an increase in the number of phage present. This procedure can be carried out several times in succession, to bulk up the number of phage enormously. Note, though, that it does not increase the number of *different* sequences that are cloned. Sometimes it may do the reverse. Phage carrying certain inserts may replicate more slowly than others. They will therefore be replicated fewer times during amplification and will as a result become underrepresented. In extreme cases, they may be lost completely, so the more times a library is amplified, the less representative it may get.

3.3.3 *In vivo* cloning in lambda

It is important to point out that lambda (and some other phages) can be used for cloning purposes without our having recourse to restriction enzymes. Induction of a lambda lysogen sometimes leads to aberrant excision of the phage from the *E. coli* chromosome. A molecule containing part of the phage DNA and part of the adjacent sequence is excised, rather than a single phage genome. Although the excised molecule itself may not contain all the phage genes for head proteins, tail proteins, and so on, these genes are still present in the cell, and the proteins will be produced. This results in the packaging of the phage, which now carry *E. coli* DNA replacing some of the phage DNA. Because of the limits on the size of molecules that can be packaged, phage particles that have acquired significant amounts of flanking sequence must have lost some phage sequence. These phage particles are called *transducing phage*; under the appropriate conditions, they can be selected and harvested, and their DNA can be obtained. Lambda is a *specialized transducing phage*, as it has a preferred site of integration into the *E. coli* chromosome (the *attachment site*) and will therefore preferentially produce transducing phage for genes near that site. If the attachment site is deleted, though, the phage can integrate elsewhere, at *secondary attachment sites*, and transduce other genes. Any phage that can acquire chromosomal DNA (not necessarily by direct integration) can be used in transduction. Phages that do not preferentially transduce particular regions of the genome are called *generalized transducing phages*. The F factor can also be used for transduction, since it can integrate and excise, at times aberrantly, from the genome to produce an F'. This process is often called *sexduction*. Both transduction and sexduction have proved enormously useful in obtaining *E. coli* genes. For more information, consult textbooks of classical bacterial genetics.

3. 3. 4 Lambda ZAP

The lambda ZAP vector is based on bacteriophage lambda but contains within it a region that can be excised *in vivo* to form one of the Bluescript plasmids (see Section 3.2.4). This is shown in Figure 3.13. The Bluescript region, which also contains the cloning sites, is flanked by two filamentous phage replication signals, the f1 *initiator* and the f1 *terminator*. The initiator is recognized by the gene II protein that is produced from a suitable helper phage. It is nicked, and synthesis of a single strand is initiated. Replication proceeds unidirectionally from this site through the Bluescript region until the terminator is reached, at which point nicking takes place again. The single-stranded sequence that is generated is then circularized *in vivo* to form a covalently closed single-stranded circular molecule, which can then be converted into a double-stranded molecule by cellular DNA synthesis.

The double-stranded molecule that has been generated is the Bluescript plasmid and can be replicated as a plasmid from the ColEI origin of replication. Alternatively, in the continued presence of helper phage it can be used to synthesize single-stranded DNA, since it also contains an f1 origin of replication (which is a hybrid between the two origin sequences in the original lambda ZAP). The single-stranded DNA can also be packaged using the coat proteins produced by helper phage. As with Bluescript, the presence of an insert is detected by inactivation of *lacZ'*. So lambda ZAP can be used to construct a phage library, containing inserts up to 10 kb. Once a suitable phage has been selected from the library, that phage is used to infect *E. coli* cells that are co-infected with the f1 helper phage. This results in Bluescript plasmid excision and packaging as single-stranded DNA. After a few hours' growth, the excised and packaged DNA is recovered. It is then used to reinfect *E. coli*. On entering *E. coli*, it is converted to double-stranded DNA by the cell, giving rise to $amp^r lacZ^-$ colonies, and is maintained as a double-stranded plasmid. This procedure has in effect allowed subcloning from the lambda phage directly into a plasmid *in vivo*. Otherwise, this would have to be done much more laboriously by excision of the insert from the phage using restriction endonucleases, followed by ligation into suitably cut vector.

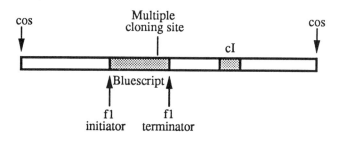

Figure 3.13 Lambda ZAP.

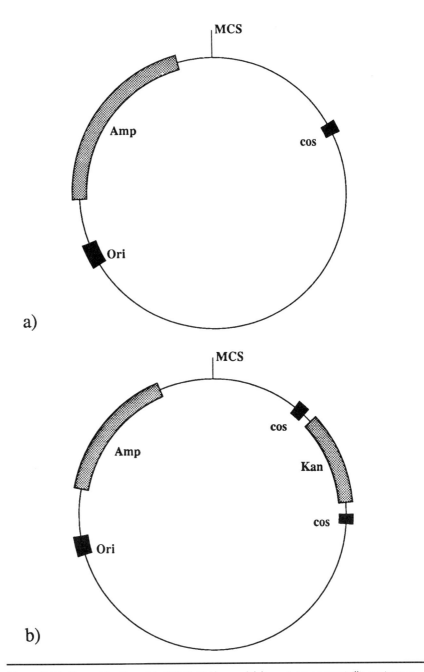

Figure 3.14 **Cosmids.** Cosmid pJB8 (5.4 kb), panel (**a**), contains an ampicillin resistance gene, an *E. coli* origin of replication, a multiple cloning site (MCS), and a *cos* site. Cosmid c2RB (6.8 kb), panel (**b**), contains a second *cos* site (and an additional selectable marker).

3. 4   COSMIDS

Cosmids can be regarded as lambda replacement vectors from which even more phage DNA has been deleted to leave only the *cos* packaging site. They also contain a plasmid origin of replication. None of the coat protein genes is left, so although cosmids can be packaged *in vitro*, once they are inside an *E. coli* cell, they cannot generate more phage and can therefore propagate only as plasmids. They cannot give rise to plaques. For this reason, some other selectable marker must be used to indicate their presence, and this is usually a beta-lactamase gene for ampicillin resistance. Entry of DNA into the host cell is therefore selected not by the formation of a plaque on a lawn, but by the formation of colonies on plates containing ampicillin. Cosmids are, in effect, bacterial plasmids that happen to be able to be packaged into phage coats for easy delivery.

The procedure for inserting DNA into cosmids is very similar to the one used with lambda. Cosmids are much smaller than lambda phage. For example, pJB8 (shown in Figure 3.14a) is only 5.4 kb. However, the same minimum-size condition for packaging and delivery to *E. coli* pertains. Hence, the only cosmids that can be successfully packaged, delivered, and form ampicillin-resistant colonies are those that have acquired large inserts. There is therefore a selection for the acquisition of large inserts, and this is the main advantage of cosmids. Typically, they will accept inserts of 35–45 kb. They are therefore very popular for the construction of genomic libraries (see Section 4.2). A drawback is that once the cosmids are inside the *E. coli* cell, there is no longer any size selection, and partial deletion may take place. Some cosmids contain two *cos* site, (e.g., c2RB, shown in Figure 3.14b). This makes it unnecessary to ensure concatemer formation before packaging (which would otherwise be necessary, as with lambda phage), because each molecule already has a pair of *cos* sites.

3. 5 BACTERIOPHAGE P1

Although the use of cosmids allows molecules up to 40 kb or so to be cloned, it is often desirable to be able to clone even larger fragments. The use of bacteriophage P1 may be useful for this purpose, as its head can accommodate some 110–115 kb. The vectors used are complex as a consequence of the packaging process, which is not as simple as the process with lambda. As with lambda vectors, the packaging constraints impose a size selection on the recombinants. Packaging of recombinant DNA is carried out *in vitro*, and the vectors will generally accept between 75 and 95 kb.

CHAPTER

4

Making
Libraries

4.1 INTRODUCTION

We encountered the concept of a library – a collection of random DNA clones –
in Section 2.1. Having learned about cloning in bacteriophage lambda and its
derivatives, we are now in a position to look in more detail at making libraries.

Libraries can conveniently be divided into two categories: genomic
libraries, which are made from the total genomic DNA of an organism, and
cDNA libraries, which are made from DNA copies of its RNA sequences. We
will look first at how these two types of library are made. Sometimes, though,
it is useful to be able to make a more specialized genomic or cDNA library,
enriched for particular sequences, so we will look at how they are made, too.
The library we looked at in Section 2.1 was a plasmid library. It was represented by a large number of colonies on a plate, each containing a plasmid with
a defined insert. We can also use a phage vector; handling large numbers of
phages is often more convenient than handling large numbers of plasmids.
When using phage, we get a collection of plaques on a lawn of bacterial cells,
rather than colonies. Each plaque will contain a single type of phage with a
defined DNA insert. With cosmids, the library will again be colonies on
a plate.

4. 2   GENOMIC LIBRARIES

4. 2. 1   Principles

A genomic library contains all the sequences present in the genome of an organism. Clearly, the larger the insert of genomic DNA in each recombinant, the lower the number of recombinants needed to represent the organism's genome completely. (The relationship between genome size, insert size, and the number of members needed for the library is discussed in more detail in Section 5.2.6.) For most purposes it is therefore best to use vectors that will accept large inserts. This effectively means lambda replacement vectors, such as EMBL4 (shown in Figure 3.11), or cosmid vectors, such as pJB8 and c2RB (shown in Figure 3.14). Yeast artificial chromosomes, which are discussed in Section 9.4.6, are increasingly widely used, as they can accept inserts even larger than those accepted by cosmids. For small genomes, lambda insertional vectors or plasmids may be suitable.

4. 2. 2   The procedure

1. The key to generating a high quality library usually lies in the preparation of the insert DNA. The first step is the isolation of genomic DNA. The procedures vary widely according to the organism under study and will not be discussed here. Care should be taken to avoid physical damage to the DNA so that it is of as high a molecular weight and as free of nicks as possible. If the intention is to prepare a nuclear DNA library, it is often sufficient to use total DNA, ignoring whatever DNA is present in the mitochondria or chloroplasts, as there is usually much more nuclear than organellar material. If the aim is to make an organelle genomic library, it would be wise to purify the organelles away from the nuclei first, and then prepare DNA from them.

2. The DNA is then fragmented to a size suitable for ligation into the vector, say 20–25 kb for EMBL4. As discussed in Section 1.2.1, this could be done by complete digestion with a restriction endonuclease, but a large number of sequences would not be represented intact (or might not be represented at all) in a library made this way. It is much better to use partial digestion with a frequently cutting enzyme to generate a random collection of fragments with a suitable size distribution. Once prepared, the fragments are often treated with phosphatase to remove terminal phosphate groups. This ensures that separate pieces of insert DNA cannot be ligated together before they are ligated into the vector. Ligation of separate fragments is undesirable, as it would generate clones containing noncontiguous DNA, and we would have with no way of knowing where the joint lay. Note that this is a different use of phosphatase from the one encountered earlier, in which the *vector* (rather than the *insert)* was treated with phosphatase to prevent self-ligation.

3. The vector is prepared.

4. Vector and insert are mixed, ligated, packaged (if appropriate), and so on, as described in Section 3.2.2.

5. If necessary, the library is amplified (Section 3.3.2). Libraries using lambda as the cloning vector are usually kept as a stock of packaged phage. Samples of this can then be plated out on an appropriate host when needed. Libraries constructed in plasmid vectors are kept as collections of plasmid-containing cells or as naked DNA that can be transformed into host cells when needed. With storage, naked DNA may be degraded. Larger molecules are more likely to be degraded than smaller ones, so larger recombinants will be selectively lost, and the average insert size will fall.

4. 3 cDNA Libraries

4. 3. 1 Principles

For cDNA libraries, we produce DNA copies of the RNA sequences (usually the mRNA) of an organism and clone them. Such libraries are particularly useful, because they represent not just the collection of expressed sequences from that organism, but those sequences after any posttranscriptional modification, such as the removal of introns. Comparison of cDNA sequences with genomic DNA sequences allows the determination of the positions of introns, polyadenylation sites, and so forth. The cDNA molecules to be cloned are often no more than a few kilobases long, so plasmid vectors may well be suitable. However, lambda insertion vectors, such as lambda gt11, are very widely used, as they have advantages for the subsequent screening process (see Section 5.2.2). For a long time, cDNA cloning was regarded as being particularly difficult, and it was notoriously hard to generate *full-length* cDNA (i.e., cDNA molecules corresponding to the entire length of the RNA species). Things were made much easier by the development of the RNaseH technique described in Section 4.3.3. The earlier techniques (involving self-priming, or tailing and priming) will also be mentioned briefly, since many important experiments made use of them.

The approach adopted depends in the initial stages on whether or not the RNA species for which cDNA is required are polyadenylated at their 3' ends. Most eukaryotic cytoplasmic mRNAs are polyadenylated. Those that are not include those for histones, some organelle mRNAs (e.g., those from chloroplasts and plant mitochondria), bacterial mRNAs, and stable mRNAs, such as ribosomal RNAs.

4. 3. 2 Polyadenylated RNA

Polyadenylated RNA (polyA$^+$ RNA) can be separated from other RNAs by fractionation on oligo-dT cellulose; that is, cellulose (acting as a solid-phase support) to which short oligonucleotides composed entirely of deoxyT residues have been covalently attached via the hydroxyl groups of the cellulose. Usually, a solution containing the RNA is passed through a column of oligo-dT cellulose. The polyA tail of the RNA forms hydrogen bonds with the oligo-dT, and polyA$^+$ RNA is therefore retained by the column. After washing all non-specifically bound RNA from the column, the polyA$^+$ RNA is eluted with a low-salt buffer. (High salt concentrations stabilize nucleic acid hybridization, low salt concentrations weaken it.) Preparation of good quality polyA$^+$ RNA is probably the most important part of cDNA cloning, and it is made especially difficult by the fact that RNA is a particularly labile molecule (much more so than DNA, because the 2'-hydroxyl group of the ribose ring increases its reactivity), necessitating careful precautions against degradation. These usually include baking all glassware and treatment with ribonuclease inhibitors. Not only is RNA particularly labile, many ribonucleases are very stable, and some can be boiled with little subsequent loss of activity.

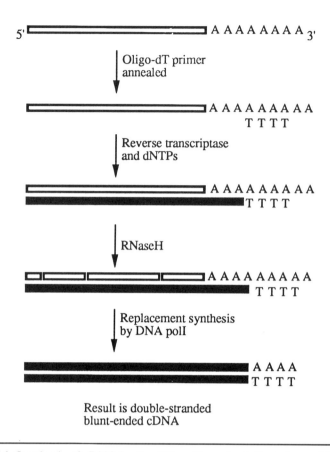

$5'$ ▭▭▭▭▭ A A A A A A A $_{3'}$

Oligo-dT primer
annealed

▭▭▭▭ A A A A A A A A
T T T T

Reverse transcriptase
and dNTPs

▭▭▭▭ A A A A A A A A
▬▬▬▬ T T T T

RNaseH

▭▯▭▭ A A A A A A A A
▬▬▬▬ T T T T

Replacement synthesis
by DNA polI

▬▬▬▬ A A A A
▬▬▬▬ T T T T

Result is double-stranded
blunt-ended cDNA

Figure 4.1 **Synthesis of cDNA by the RNaseH method**. Shaded material is DNA, the rest RNA.

4. 3. 3 cDNA synthesis

1. The RNaseH method. In this method, a complementary DNA strand is synthesized using reverse transcriptase (Section 1.3.2) to make an RNA:DNA duplex, and the RNA strand is then nicked and replaced by DNA (Figure 4.1). The first step is to anneal a chemically synthesized oligo-dT primer to the 3' polyA tail of the RNA. The primer is typically 10–15 residues long and primes synthesis of the first DNA strand with reverse transcriptase and deoxyribonucleotides. This leaves an RNA:DNA duplex, and the next step is to replace the RNA strand with a DNA strand. The difficulty is finding a way to prime synthesis using the DNA strand as template. Annealing oligo-dA to the oligo-dT incorporated during synthesis of the first strand would be no use; the oligo-dT is at the 5' end of the DNA template molecule, but synthesis must start at the 3' end. There is no way to predict the sequence at the 3' end. However, we can use as a primer the RNA that is already attached to the DNA. In practice, this is done by treating the RNA:DNA duplex with a low concentration of RNaseH, together with DNA polI and deoxyribonucleotides. The RNase nicks the RNA, leaving free 3'-hydroxyl groups, and DNA can then be made using these as primers. (Remember that DNA synthesis *in vivo* uses RNA primers with free 3'-hydroxyls.) As DNA chains are synthesized, any molecules that are base-paired to the template further down are displaced or degraded by the polymerase. Eventually this leaves a DNA:DNA duplex, perhaps with a small region of RNA including any 5' cap at one end (which doesn't seem to interfere with subsequent cloning). We will next look at the *self-priming* method of generating cDNA and then see how cDNA generated by either the RNaseH method or the self-priming method can be ligated into a vector.

2. The self-priming method. This represents another approach to the problem of converting a DNA:RNA duplex into a DNA:DNA one. It is shown in Figure 4.2. An RNA:DNA duplex is obtained as before. It is then treated with dilute sodium hydroxide, which hydrolyses the RNA. (DNA is not hydrolysed by dilute alkali, because of the lack of the 2'-hydroxyl groups.) This leaves a single DNA strand. As before, the oligo-dT cannot be exploited for second-strand synthesis, because it is at the wrong end of the first strand. The self-priming approach relies on the chance occurrence of complementarity between a region near the 3' end of the molecule and a region further to the 5' end. This would allow the molecule to form a "hairpin" loop. The base-paired region that results, with its free 3'-hydroxyl, is now able to act as a primer for DNA synthesis. This completes the second DNA strand. The loop must be removed, and this is done by treatment with S1 nuclease, which degrades single-stranded regions such as the loop. The result is a double-stranded, blunt-ended molecule, which can now be inserted into vector, as described before, with blunt-ended ligation, linkers, or tailing.

Clearly this technique has several important disadvantages. There is no intrinsic reason why there should be complementarity between the 3' end and other parts of the first strand. So priming may not be able to take place at all and may well be very inefficient. Furthermore, at least some of the first strand is lost in this process (indicated in Figure 4.2), which is a major factor contributing to the difficulty of getting full-length cDNA clones using this technique.

Both the RNaseH and the self-priming procedures ultimately generate a double-stranded, blunt-ended DNA molecule. It must now be attached to the vector. This could be done by blunt-ended ligation or by the addition of linkers, digestion with the relevant enzyme, and ligation into vector as described in Section 2.4.1. (Remember the need for methylase treatment if linkers are to be used.) A less common option is homopolymer tailing, shown in Figure 4.3. This approach exploits the enzyme terminal (deoxynucleotidyl) transferase, which can polymerize nucleotides onto the 3' end of an existing DNA molecule without the need for a template. (This enzyme caused some confusion in early work on the enzymology of DNA synthesis, as it led to the erroneous belief that physiological DNA replication does not require a template.) In principle, the approach relies on the addition of complementary tails to cDNA and vector. Treatment of the cDNA with terminal transferase and dCTP leads to the polymerization of several C residues (typically 20 or so) to the 3'-hydroxyl at each end. Treatment of the vector with terminal transferase and dGTP leads to the incorporation of several G residues onto the ends of the vector. (Alternatively, dATP and dTTP can be used.) The vector and cDNA can now anneal, and the base-paired region is often so extensive that treatment with DNA ligase is unnecessary. In fact, there may be gaps rather than nicks at the vector–insert boundaries, but these are repaired by physiological processes once the recombinant molecules have been introduced into a host.

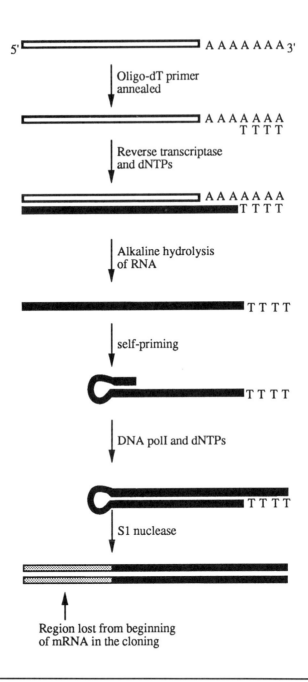

Figure 4.2 **Synthesis of cDNA by the self-priming method**. Black regions represent DNA, open regions RNA. The shaded region represents material that is not represented in the final cDNA because of the loss of material in the self-priming.

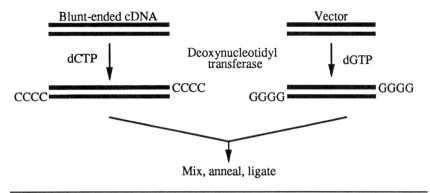

Figure 4.3 **Homopolymer tailing.**

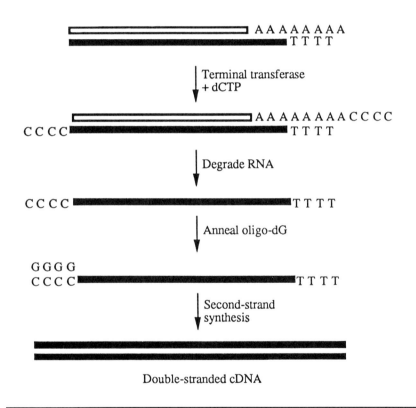

Figure 4.4 **Homopolymer tailing to provide a priming site for second-strand synthesis.** Shaded material is DNA, the rest RNA.

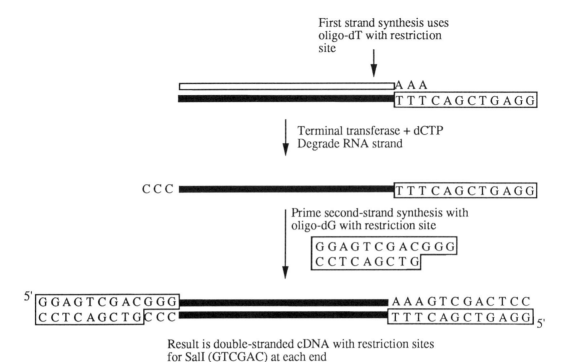

Figure 4.5 **Modification of homopolymer tailing, incorporating restriction sites.** The protocol is essentially the same as in Figure 4.4, except that the oligo-dT and oligo-dG primers also contain *Sal*I restriction sites. For clarity, the primers are shown boxed.

3. Tailing and priming. There are several variations on this approach, which also uses the enzyme terminal transferase. The approach is used for synthesis of the second strand and allows incorporation of restriction sites for insertion of cDNA into the vector. An example is shown in Figure 4.4. Instead of using terminal transferase to add tails to a DNA:DNA duplex, we use it to add tails to the RNA:DNA duplex. It can polymerize nucleotides onto the 3'-hydroxyl of both an RNA molecule as well as a DNA molecule, but the important point is that after tailing, the DNA strand of the duplex has a known sequence at its 3' end – an oligomer of whichever nucleotide was used in the tailing reaction. Typically, dCTP is used. A complementary oligomer (synthesized chemically) can now be annealed and used as a primer to direct second-strand synthesis. This oligomer (and also the one used for first-strand synthesis) may additionally incorporate a restriction site, so that linkers do not need to be added. Use of these oligonucleotides is shown in Figure 4.5. The oligo-dT primer is modified to contain a *Sal*I site (-GTCGAC-). The 3' end of the newly synthesized first cDNA strand is tailed with C's. An oligo-dG primer, again preceded by a *Sal*I site within a short double-stranded region of the oligonucleotide, is then used for second-strand synthesis. Note that this method requires the use of an oligonucleotide containing a double-stranded region. Such oligonucleotides are made by synthesizing the two strands separately and then allowing them to anneal to one another.

4. 3. 4   Nonpolyadenylated RNA

If the RNA is not polyadenylated, we cannot use oligo-dT to prime from the polyA tail. Instead, a collection of chemically synthesized oligonucleotides of random sequence are used. These are usually hexamers and are produced by oligomerization of equal quantities of mixed A, G, C, and T residues, so that all possible hexameric sequences should be present. The hexamers will therefore be able to bind throughout the length of the RNA molecule to prime synthesis of the first DNA strand. Synthesis of the second DNA strand is conveniently carried out with RNaseH and DNA polymerase I, as described in Section 4.3.3.

4. 4   SPECIALIZED LIBRARIES

It is often helpful to make libraries that are enriched for a particular fraction of genomic DNA or cDNA. This may be the case if we are trying to clone a particular gene, for example, and have some limited information about, say, chromosomal location.

4. 4. 1   Shelves

Sometimes we know the size of the restriction fragment on which a particular gene is located. For example, this information may be acquired by probing a Southern blot of digested genomic DNA with a suitable sequence, such as an oligonucleotide probe, and measuring the size(s) of restriction fragment(s) that hybridize. Once the size of the relevant restriction fragment is known, another digest of genomic DNA is then carried out with the same enzyme and electrophoresed, and DNA fragments of approximately that size are recovered from the gel. They are then cloned into a suitable vector. Because the fragments to be cloned are likely to be smaller than the random 20-kb fragments used in making full genomic libraries, a plasmid vector is often suitable. The collection of recombinants generated is frequently called a *shelf,* as it is a subsection of a library.

4. 4. 2   RNA selection

1. Tissue type. Any cDNA library is likely to represent only a fraction of the RNA species of any one organism, determined by the particular type, developmental stage, physiological state, and so on, of the tissue from which the RNA was isolated. The library would therefore be expected to contain cDNAs for the general "housekeeping" genes and for those genes whose expression is specific to that particular tissue. If we are interested in obtaining the cDNA for a specific protein, it is wise to use a cDNA library from a tissue with a lot of RNA for that protein relative to other RNAs; in other words, we should use a cDNA library from tissue producing large amounts of the protein.

2. RNA fractionation. We have seen that fractionation on an oligo-dT–cellulose column can be used to separate polyA$^+$ RNA from polyA$^-$ RNA, such as rRNA, prior to the creation of the cDNA library. It may be useful to fractionate the mRNA further to obtain a population enriched for the RNA for a particular protein. The procedure outlined here requires the availability of antibodies to the protein. The RNA (usually after the separation on oligo-dT cellulose) is fractionated by size using sucrose density gradient centrifugation. The RNA is applied to the top of a pre-poured gradient, and during centrifugation the larger molecules move down the centrifuge tube faster. The contents of the tube are then fractionated (usually by piercing the bottom and collecting individual drops or volumes). Each fraction will contain a different size-class of mRNA. A sample of each fraction is then translated *in vitro*. This is done either in an extract of wheat germ or in a lysate of rabbit reticulocyte cells. Both these preparations contain the necessary ribosomes, tRNAs, and other components to translate the added mRNA with a low background of translation products from endogenous mRNA. At least one radioactively labelled amino acid is added with the mRNA, so that all the polypeptides subsequently synthesized will be radioactively labelled (and therefore can be detected in very low quantities and also distinguished from all the polypeptides present initially in the lysate or extract).

The polypeptides produced by synthesis from the added mRNA are then analysed with the antibodies. The latter are added to each reaction tube and will bind to the corresponding protein wherever it has been produced. The antibodies and any bound protein can then be precipitated and recovered. Rather than relying on simple precipitation of the antibody-antigen complex, it is wise to add something that will bind antibodies but can easily be precipitated. Protein A–Sepharose is convenient for this purpose. Protein A occurs on the outside of *Staphylococcus aureus* cells and binds IgG antibodies. It will therefore bind to the antibodies added to the translation products, and the antibodies will in turn be bound to the protein of interest (in any tubes where it has been produced). Because the Protein A is also attached to Sepharose beads (covalently coupled using cyanogen bromide), it can be pelleted and collected by centrifugation along with the antibodies and any bound antigen. (As an alternative to Protein A–Sepharose, intact *S. aureus* cells can be used.) The Protein A–Sepharose pellet recovered from each tube is then denatured and electrophoresed in an SDS-polyacrylamide gel, and the location and amount of radioactive polypeptides are determined by fluorography or autoradiography. RNA fractions highly enriched for the mRNA of interest are identified as those from which large amounts of radioactive protein were precipitated by the antibodies and Protein A. These fractions are then used for the subsequent cDNA cloning to generate a library enriched for the cDNAs for particular mRNAs. Note that such a library is *not* representative of the total mRNA population from that tissue type.

4. 4. 3 Chromosome sorting

It may be that a gene of interest has been mapped to a particular chromosome. A DNA library produced not from the entire genome, but from just that chromosome, will therefore be enriched for the gene of interest. Separation of intact chromosomes can be achieved using PFGE (see Section 1.6.5), but for cloning purposes a fluorescence-activated sorter is often used. The chromosomes should be in the metaphase state, because they will then be highly condensed and not too difficult to handle. They are isolated by gentle lysis of dividing cells. They are then stained with a fluorescent dye, such as ethidium bromide (or a combination of dyes), and passed through the sorter, as shown in Figure 4.6. Each chromosome is driven by an electric field through a laser beam, which causes the dye to fluoresce. The amount of fluorescence is dependent on the amount of

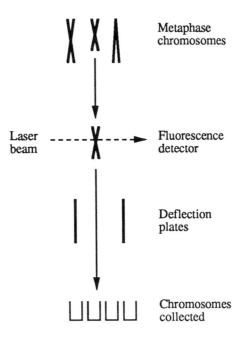

Metaphase
chromosomes

Laser
beam

Fluorescence
detector

Deflection
plates

Chromosomes
collected

Figure 4.6 **Chromosome sorting.**

dye bound to the chromosome, and this in turn depends upon the size of the chromosome. The amount of fluorescence is measured by a suitable detector, and the sorter uses the measurements to identify particular chromosomes. Application of an electric field across deflection plates, through which the chromosomes pass next, allows individual chromosomes to be deflected and collected. Once enough material has been collected, it can be deproteinized and used to prepare a library for that chromosome.

4. 4. 4   Microdissection

If a gene has been mapped to a particular chromosome or to a region on it, it may be possible to use microdissection to obtain material for cloning. Stained chromosomes are examined in a light microscope, and whole chromosomes or appropriate regions are removed with the aid of a micro-manipulator. The material is then collected in a pipette and used for cloning as before.

4. 4. 5   Deletion enrichment

Deletion enrichment is appropriate when a mutant is available from which the gene of interest has been deleted. The method, summarized in Figure 4.7, allows enrichment for those sequences that are present in the wild type, but deleted from the mutant (shaded in Figure 4.7). The first step is to prepare DNA from the individual with the deletion (call it Type A) and to sonicate it. This will produce fragments with nonspecific ends (Section 1.2.3). DNA is also prepared from a wild-type individual (call it Type B) and partially digested with an enzyme such as *Sau*3A, so all the molecules generated will have identical ends.

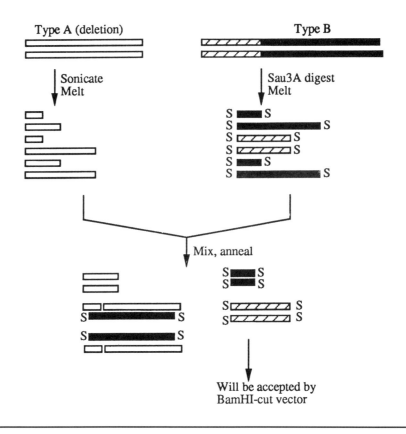

Figure 4.7 Deletion enrichment. Open boxes indicate DNA present in the Type A cells (from which some DNA has been deleted). Black material indicates the equivalent sequences in Type B cells. Shaded material represents DNA that is present in Type B cells only. S = *Sau*3A sticky end.

Each DNA preparation is melted. They are then mixed together and allowed to reanneal. Three classes of molecule will result, as shown in Figure 4.7. One will be produced by the annealing of two Type A molecules, one will be produced by the annealing of two Type B molecules, and the third will be produced by the annealing of a Type A and a Type B molecule. However, the sequences that are deleted from the Type A individuals will be present *only* in Type B molecules and therefore will form only Type B:Type B duplexes. These are also the only molecules with "clonable" (i.e., *Sau*3A) ends. So cloning of the molecules produced after annealing into a *Sau*3A-accepting vector will result in preferential cloning of the sequences present in Type B but absent from Type A. (Use of an excess of the Type A DNA over Type B will increase the enrichment, as there will generally be less likelihood that B:B duplexes will form, and Types A:A and A:B will predominate.)

4. 4. 6 Subtractive hybridization

The subtractive hybridization procedure (Figure 4.8) is in a sense analogous to deletion enrichment, but it works at the RNA level, whereas deletion enrich-

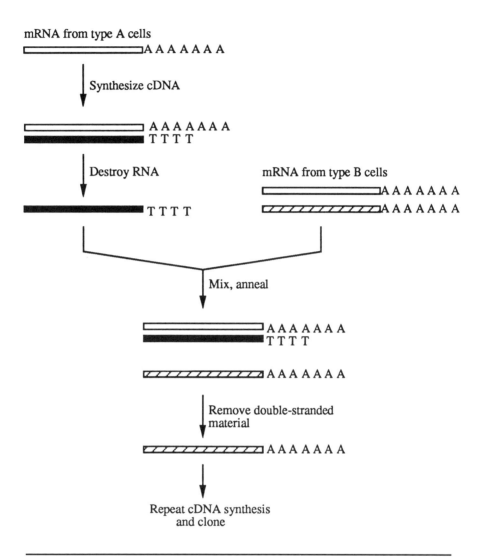

mRNA from type A cells

Synthesize cDNA

Destroy RNA

mRNA from type B cells

Mix, anneal

Remove double-stranded material

Repeat cDNA synthesis and clone

Figure 4.8 **Subtractive hybridization.** Open boxes indicate mRNA present in both cell types. Shaded material is mRNA present only in one cell type (Type B). Black material is DNA synthesized from mRNA.

ment is carried out with DNA. Subtractive hybridization allows enrichment for RNA species that are absent from one cell type (Type A) but present in another (Type B). The difference in occurrence of RNA might be due to a mutation in Type A cells that abolishes the production of the mRNA, or it might simply be due to the treatment of Type B cells in a way that induces the synthesis of the mRNA.

The mRNA is isolated from both cell types, and a single strand of complementary DNA is synthesized with an oligo-dT primer on the RNA from the Type A cells. The RNA strand of these RNA:DNA duplexes is then destroyed, leaving single complementary DNA strands. These are then mixed with the

RNA from Type B cells, and annealing is allowed to take place. The RNA species that are unique to Type B cells (shaded in Figure 4.8) will not be able to anneal to the cDNA from Type A cells (because the Type A cells did not contain that RNA) and will remain as single strands. After annealing, the material is passed down a hydroxyapatite column, which binds more tightly to double-stranded nucleic acids than to single-stranded. The single-stranded RNA is then recovered and used for cloning.

CHAPTER

5

Screening Libraries

5. 1 INTRODUCTION

So far, we have seen how libraries can be constructed using plasmids, phages, and other vectors in *E. coli*. But it is not enough simply to be able to clone DNA at random. It is necessary to be able then to identify members of a library that contain a piece of DNA with particular properties. Finding those members of the library is called *screening*. Most often, we screen libraries for sequences with a particular coding function – to find the gene or cDNA for a particular protein. There are many different strategies for doing that, and we will look at those first. Sometimes libraries are screened for DNA with a particular function other than a coding one, such as the ability to initiate transcription. We will look at those techniques too.

5. 2 SCREENING FOR CODING FUNCTION

5. 2. 1 Principles

We will assume throughout this section that the aim is to find library members encoding a particular protein. Screening for sequences encoding RNAs such as rRNAs is also possible, using similar approaches. The techniques can be divided into three classes:

    a. those that rely on expression of the coding function *in vivo*,

    b. those that rely on nucleic acid hybridization, and

    c. those that rely on the expression of the coding function *in vitro*.

These categorizations are to some extent arbitrary – in particular, there is often overlap between the second and third approaches, as we shall see. The actual approach taken will depend on which kind of library is to be screened and what is available for the selection process (nucleic acid probes, antibodies, etc.). How to choose the right approach is discussed in more detail in Section 5.2.6. The techniques are most commonly used for screening libraries constructed in *E. coli*, but they can generally also be used to screen libraries constructed in other hosts, such as cultured mammalian cells.

5. 2. 2   Expression of the coding function *in vivo*

1. Direct selection for insert function. This approach is possible if the cloned gene can be expressed in the host and can complement a suitable mutant strain. For example, suppose the aim is to clone the gene for the transport protein required for the uptake of a particular sugar by *E. coli*. The first requirement in this approach is to isolate by conventional microbiological techniques (or to obtain from a culture collection) a strain carrying a mutation in that gene, so that the strain cannot take up the sugar and is therefore unable to grow on medium containing the sugar as the sole carbon source. A library is then made from a wild-type strain and introduced into the mutant strain by transformation, phage infection, or whatever means is appropriate. After selection for the acquisition of recombinant molecules, selection is then imposed for complementation of the mutation – in this case, for the ability to grow on medium containing the sugar as the sole carbon source. Individuals that are able to do that are likely to have acquired a wild-type copy of the relevant gene from the library.

This approach (summarized in Figure 5.1) need not be restricted to the identification of recombinants carrying nutritional markers. As long as a mutant strain can be obtained and complementation of the mutant can be selected, the approach can be tried. However, there are a number of requirements and possible problems.

DETAILED UNDERSTANDING OF THE POSSIBLE CAUSES OF COMPLEMENTATION IS NEEDED. Suppose (as is indeed often the case) there were a number of different proteins able to transport the sugar. A mutant that was deficient in transport could therefore be complemented by any of a number of different genes from the library. Before using this approach, it is therefore important to be aware of alternative means by which the initial mutant phenotype might be complemented.

THE MUTANT HOST MUST HAVE A LOW REVERSION RATE. The proportion of recombinants that carry the gene of interest – and are therefore able to complement the host mutation – is likely to be low and may be lower than the spontaneous reversion rate of the mutation used. A consequence of that would be that most of the individuals selected would be the products not of complementation, but simply of reversion of the original mutation and would not be of interest.

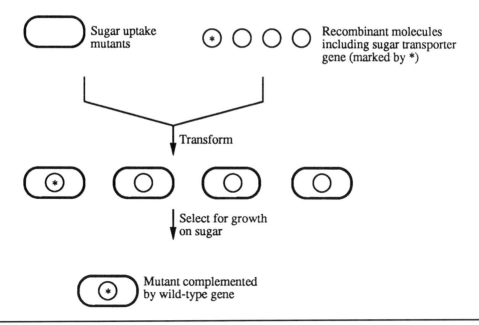

Figure 5.1 Selection for functional complementation. * = a gene for uptake of a particular sugar. In a sugar uptake mutant background, only the transformant carrying that gene can grow when the sugar is the sole source of carbon.

However, the mutation used should affect one gene only, so mutant strains with large deletions (or polar mutations, which affect several genes) would not be suitable, even though they may have a low reversion rate.

OTHER FEATURES OF THE HOST GENOTYPE MAY BE IMPORTANT. It is not sufficient for the host just to contain a mutation in the gene of interest. The genetic background is also important. As with other hosts (Section 2.2.3), the one used here should be deficient in restriction enzymes; otherwise, the incoming DNA may be degraded unless it has been protected by methylation. The host should also be deficient in recombination, or the incoming DNA may become rearranged or integrated into the host chromosome (and would then be very difficult to recover). Many of the mutant strains used in more classical microbiological analysis do not have these characteristics, so they would need to be altered suitably. Depending on the strains involved, this may well be a relatively straightforward exercise in traditional bacterial genetics.

THE GENE MAY NOT BE EXPRESSED EFFICIENTLY. This is particularly likely to be the case if the gene comes from a different species from the one in which the selection is carried out (in which case the selection is said to be *heterologous* rather than *homologous*), because the sequences required for expression may also differ between species. If the gene being screened for is prokaryotic, and even if it comes from the same species, it may still not be expressed if it is such a long way from its promoter that the promoter is unlikely to be present in the insert; cDNA sequences are unlikely to have any of the associated expression sequences at all. It may be possible to circumvent some of these problems by the use of *expression vectors* (see Section 8.3.4), which are designed to allow the controlled expression of any genes cloned into them. Any introns present will not be excised after transcription in the prokaryotic host, so even with expression vectors the approach is not generally suitable for use with eukaryotic genomic libraries.

IF EXPRESSED, THE PROTEIN MAY BE NONFUNCTIONAL. This problem may arise in heterologous selection, especially if the protein has to interact physically with others for its function, because these interactions are less likely to occur efficiently in a heterologous situation.

These difficulties may seem so great that the technique is unlikely to work, although very often only a partial restoration of function is needed to identify the desired constructs satisfactorily. In fact, this approach does have two important advantages. One is the fact that there is no need to have antibodies available to the product of the gene in question or to have any prior information on DNA or amino acid sequence (which many other techniques require). The other advantage is that direct selection on a plate allows a very large number of recombinants to be screened quickly and easily.

Another approach to screening for insert function (although it is not strictly complementation) is to use *Xenopus* oocytes. DNA from collections of recombinants is transcribed *in vitro*, and the transcription products are microinjected into oocytes. The RNA is translated within the oocytes, which are then screened for the function of interest. This approach has proved particularly useful for finding clones for membrane proteins with physiological functions that can be easily identified, such as the transport of ions or metabolites.

2. Ligand binding by the expressed protein. In this approach, the expression of a cloned gene is detected not by the phenotype it confers, but by the ability of the protein it encodes to bind particular ligands. Very often, screening of libraries for ligand binding is done immunochemically, with antibodies. However, if the sequence we are screening for encodes a receptor protein, we may be able to use the receptor's ligand instead of antibodies. Or, if we are screening for sequences encoding proteins able to bind a specific DNA sequence, we can use that DNA. The procedure for immunochemical screening of plasmid libraries, summarized in Figure 5.2, is as follows:

  a. A nitrocellulose membrane is placed onto the plate containing the colonies to be screened and then peeled off. This brings some of the bacteria from each colony with it. (The original plate can then be reincubated to allow the colonies to regenerate.) The membrane is then exposed to chloroform vapour to permeabilize the colonies and is soaked in a lysis buffer. Proteins from the lysed colonies adhere to the membrane.

  b. After washing the membrane and blocking nonspecific protein binding sites (usually with a suspension of dried milk powder), we incubate the membrane with the antibodies. If any members of the library are producing the relevant protein, the protein will be present on the membrane at the position corresponding to those members of the library, and the antibodies will bind to it.

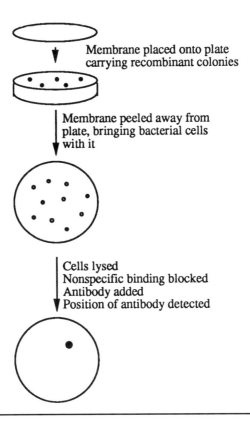

Membrane placed onto plate
carrying recombinant colonies

Membrane peeled away from
plate, bringing bacterial cells
with it

Cells lysed
Nonspecific binding blocked
Antibody added
Position of antibody detected

Figure 5.2 **Immunochemical screening of plasmid libraries**. If some other ligand
is being used, this would be substituted for the antibodies in the penultimate step.

c. The membrane is again washed. Now we can detect the position of bound
antibody. This can be done by incubation with a second antibody – one
which has been labelled for detection by chemiluminescence and will
cross-react with the first antibody – or by incubation with radiolabelled
Protein A (see Section 4.4.2), which will bind to the first antibody.
(Antibodies labelled for chemiluminescence detection are supplied commercially. They are conjugated to horseradish peroxidase, which catalyses a light-emitting reaction in the presence of appropriate substrates.)
The sites where the first antibody has been bound indicate the positions
of recombinants expressing the gene for the protein of interest. (It is
often a good idea to prepare duplicate membranes initially, so that spurious background signals can be distinguished from genuine signals that
should be seen on both membranes.) The same general procedure can
also be applied to screening phage libraries and to the use of other ligands. For the latter, you can use a radioactively labelled ligand and detect
its position autoradiographically.

The ligand-binding approach is very widely used, although it requires the
availability of antibodies or some other ligand. It is essential that the binding
activity be preserved during the processing. It also requires that only a single

protein species be necessary to bind to the ligand. If the ligand binds only to a heterodimer, then recombinants would have to produce both of the proteins to bind the ligand successfully; this is very unlikely. Screening by ligand binding also requires expression of the gene in the host. This is particularly likely to be a problem when dealing with eukaryotic genes inserted into prokaryotic hosts. The expression signals are unlikely to be functional, and in the case of cDNA, the signals are unlikely to be present anyway. The requirement for expression can be satisfied by the use of expression vectors, which are designed to give controlled expression of genes inserted into the vector. (These are discussed further in Section 8.3.4.) The presence of introns in the insert DNA is likely to pose severe problems, even if expression vectors are used, so the ligand-binding technique is largely restricted to screening cDNA libraries.

A variant of the ligand-binding approach is called *panning*. Here the ligand is immobilized on a solid-phase support and cells are passed over it. If the ligand-binding domain is exposed on the surface of any of the recombinants, they will be retained and can then be recovered. This is particularly useful for screening libraries in cultured mammalian cells, where there is no cell wall to get in the way (see Section 9.9.1). The same approach can be used with the phage display vectors described in Section 3.2.4. The phage retained in the panning will be those displaying the required protein in their coats and, therefore, incorporating the required DNA into the phage genome. Panning is unlikely to be suitable for screening libraries in *E. coli*, unless the protein product of interest is exposed on the outside of the cell.

5. 2. 3 Nucleic acid hybridization

Most of the nucleic acid hybridization screening techniques rely on one kind of experiment – the *colony lift* or *plaque lift*. Considerable variation is possible in the nature of the probe sequence, though. We will first look at the basic experiment and then discuss the kinds of probe available. We will also look at three examples of more specialized applications of this technique.

1. The *colony lift* or *plaque lift*. This technique is often called the Grunstein-Hogness technique after the people who developed it. In essence, it is an experiment to find out which members of a library contain sequences complementary to a "probe" DNA sequence. The library may be either *E. coli* colonies on a plate (in which case the experiment is called a colony lift) or plaques on a bacterial lawn (in which case it is called a plaque lift). The experiment is similar to the immunochemical screening outlined in Section 5.2.2. The technique (Figure 5.3) is as follows :

   a. A piece of a suitable membrane is laid onto the plate for a few seconds and then peeled off. It will bring with it phage particles or bacterial cells adhering to the membrane. As with immunochemical screening, it is wise to carry out the experiment with duplicate membranes to distinguish genuine signals from random background ones.

   b. The membrane is treated with sodium hydroxide to lyse bacterial cells and to denature phage proteins and the DNA.

   c. The membrane is treated with a neutralizing buffer and baked at 80°C to bind the DNA irreversibly to the membrane. UV crosslinking is some-

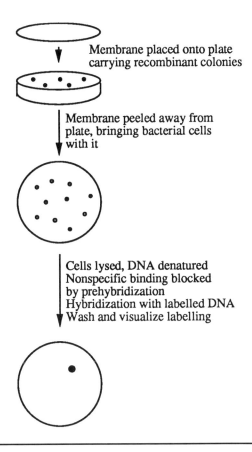

Membrane placed onto plate
carrying recombinant colonies

Membrane peeled away from
plate, bringing bacterial cells
with it

Cells lysed, DNA denatured
Nonspecific binding blocked
by prehybridization
Hybridization with labelled DNA
Wash and visualize labelling

Figure 5.3 **Colony lift**. The same procedure can be used with a phage library; instead of plasmid DNA from bacterial colonies, phage DNA will be adsorbed onto the membrane.

times used as well. The baking or crosslinking may be omitted with certain types of membrane.

d. Nonspecific DNA binding sites on the membrane are then blocked by treatment with a "prehybridization" mix containing nonlabelled DNA of nonspecific sequence (usually from salmon or herring testes or sperm). The membrane is washed, and labelled probe DNA is added and allowed to hybridize to any complementary sequences on the membrane.

e. After hybridization, the membrane is washed again, and the position of labelled probe DNA is determined. This will be by autoradiography if the probe is radioactively labelled, but other labelling and visualization techniques are available, such as chemiluminescence. (There are various labelling methods available for chemiluminescence, but commonly the probe is labelled by incorporation of fluorescein-conjugated nucleotides. Detection is by an antifluorescein antibody conjugated to horseradish peroxidase. Using appropriate substrates, this enzyme catalyses a reaction resulting in the emission of light that is detected with a photographic film.)

f. The position of bound probe DNA indicates the position of plaques or colonies containing complementary, and therefore homologous, sequences.

Originally, nitrocellulose was the preferred membrane. This binds DNA very efficiently and therefore made the technique very sensitive. However, it has the disadvantage of being very brittle and is therefore difficult to handle without breakage. Subsequently, nylon membranes were used; these are less inflammable and more durable than nitrocellulose, although they do not always offer the same sensitivity. Better sensitivity can be obtained by using derivatized nylon membranes, which bind DNA more effectively.

The precise conditions for annealing of the probe and subsequent washing are critical. The important parameters are the size of the probe, the proportions of A's, G's, C's, and T's, the ionic concentration of the hybridization buffer, and the presence (or absence) of other agents, such as formamide, which destabilize base-paired DNA. These parameters determine the maximum temperature at which the probe and its target DNA (if fully complementary) will remain base-paired. Hybridization must therefore be carried out at a temperature somewhat lower than this maximum. Carrying it out at a lower temperature still allows some mismatching between the probe and its target, so that the probe need not be a perfectly complementary sequence. This will be discussed later in this section.

The key to success in these experiments is to use a suitable probe. The following sections describe the types most commonly used.

OLIGONUCLEOTIDE PROBES. If information is already available on the amino acid sequence of the protein in question (usually obtained by direct amino-acid sequence determination of a few residues of the purified protein), it is possible to synthesize chemically an oligonucleotide that would encode that sequence. That oligonucleotide can then be used as a probe. However, because of the degeneracy of the genetic code, it will not be possible to deduce the corresponding nucleotide sequence with certainty. Although (in the "universal" code) there is only a single codon for methionine and a single codon for tryptophan, there are between two and six codons for each of the other amino acids. The best regions of amino acid sequence for constructing oligonucleotides are therefore those that are rich in methionine or tryptophan residues or, failing that, residues with only two codons. Most organisms have a preference for some codons over others for the same amino acid, so it may be possible to use this information to make an informed guess as to which of several choices is likely to be used. Otherwise, it may be necessary to have a *mixed site* in the oligonucleotide. This means that a mixture of two or more nucleotides is used in a particular cycle of oligonucleotide synthesis (see Section 1.7), and different nucleotides will be put into different molecules. The result is a mixture of oligonucleotides with slightly different sequences. An example of this is given in Figure 5.4.

If enough mixed sites are included, we can be sure that the "correct" sequence will be among those present. However, as more and more mixed sites are used, that correct sequence will come to represent a smaller and smaller proportion of the total number of sequences in the probe, and the signal generated on the autoradiograph after screening the library will get correspondingly weaker and weaker. Furthermore, the greater the number of incorrect sequences

```
T T C A T G C A A T A C C C A G G A A T G T A C C C
    T           G       T       C       C               T
                                G       G
                                T       T
```

Phe   Met   Gln   Tyr   Pro   Gly   Met   Tyr   Pro

T T C A T G C A G T A C C C C G G C A T G T A C C C

Figure 5.4 **Oligonucleotide probes.** The middle line shows a stretch of amino acid sequence. Above it is the sequence of a "mixed" oligonucleotide containing all possible sequences encoding that stretch of amino acids. Below it is a "best guess" sequence for an organism where the order of preference of nucleotides at the third codon position is C>G>A>T.

present, the more likely it is that at least one of them will be able to anneal to another sequence in the library that is unrelated to the one we want, giving rise to a consistent, but false, positive signal in the screening process. An alternative to using mixed sites is to incorporate a *neutral* base, such as inosine. This can pair (although not necessarily strongly) with all of the standard bases. Designing oligonucleotides therefore requires a careful balance between informed guesses and mixed or neutral sites.

The temperature T_m at which a short oligonucleotide (containing 18 nucleotides or fewer) will melt from its target sequence is given by the following equation:

$$T_m = (\text{number of A's and T's}) \times 2°C + (\text{number of C's and G's}) \times 4°C$$

For longer molecules,

$$T_m = 81.5 + 16.6\log_{10}[Na^+] + 0.41(\%GC) - 600/N$$

where $[Na^+]$ is the molar concentration of sodium ions, %GC is the percentage of GC base pairs in the probe, and N is its length.

Hybridization is therefore carried out at a few degrees below this temperature to ensure that probe and target can indeed hybridize. Mismatches can be allowed for by lowering the temperature still further. However, this also increases the risk of the probe's annealing to a sequence other than the true target and generating a false positive signal. It is a wise precaution, if enough amino acid sequence is available, to make two oligonucleotide probes – each for a different part of the protein sequence – and accept as genuine positives in the screening only those clones that hybridize to both oligonucleotides.

It may also be wise to use a cDNA library rather than a genomic library when screening in this way. Because cDNA libraries are enriched for coding sequences, fewer members need to be screened in order to find a suitable clone, and the risk of the probe's hybridizing to a "wrong" sequence is therefore lower.

DNA PROBES. Longer DNA sequences (referred to here as "DNA probes") are often available, and since they are longer than the oligonucleotides described, there is less danger of a spurious positive result when using them as a probe. The sequences available might be a

    a. cDNA clone. If a sequence has been isolated from a cDNA library (perhaps by oligonucleotide hybridization), it can then be used to probe a genomic library to identify genomic clones. It can also be used to reprobe the same cDNA library (or a different one) to identify more cDNA clones.

    b. genomic DNA clone. This too can be used to screen a cDNA library or a genomic one. Screening a genomic library allows the isolation of clones containing more copies of the gene (particularly useful when dealing with multigene families) or clones overlapping with the first (see "Chromosome walking" later in Section 5.2.3).

It is of course no use to screen a library by hybridization with a clone containing the same vector sequence that was used to make the library, because the vector will hybridize to all the members of the library. Either the probe must be separated from the vector, perhaps by agarose gel electrophoresis and recovery from the gel (Section 1.6.2), or the probe must be in a vector that does not have any sequence homology with the library to be screened. It is notoriously difficult to separate DNA fragments from all possible contaminating fragments in a gel, so use of a completely different vector is much more reliable. Unfortunately, so many vectors have sequences in common (such as particular drug resistance genes or particular origins of replication) that this is often difficult.

Like oligonucleotide probes, DNA probes used for screening libraries do not have to match the target sequence completely. As a rough guide, the melting temperature of a perfectly matched DNA probe is given by the same equation used for long oligonucleotide:

$$T_m = 81.5 + 16.6\log_{10}[Na^+] + 0.41(\%GC) - 600/N$$

where $[Na^+]$ is the molar concentration of sodium ions, %GC is the percentage of GC base pairs in the probe, and N is its length.

As with oligonucleotide probes, hybridization and washing when using DNA probes are usually carried out at a few degrees below this melting temperature. A 1% mismatch between the target and probe sequences lowers the melting temperature by $1°-1.5°C$, so hybridization and washing at lower temperatures can be used to allow for mismatch. The greater the degree of mismatch allowed, the less *stringent* the hybridization is said to be, and the greater the possibility of hybridization of the probe to the "wrong" clones by chance complementarity.

The ability to allow for mismatch between probe and target means that they do not have to come from the same species. If they do come from the same species, the hybridization is said to be *homologous*. If not, it is said to be *heterologous* (even though there must be homology between probe and target for hybridization to work). So once a sequence has been cloned from one species, it can be more easily obtained from other species, too.

RNA PROBES. Under some circumstances, RNA species may be used as probes. If a particular RNA can be purified, it can be used as a specific probe for the corresponding DNA species. Complete purification of particular RNAs is rarely possible, except for species such as rRNAs and tRNAs. More often a *differential hybridization* approach, sometimes called *positive-negative screening*, is adopted. This offers a way of identifying clones for RNAs that are present in one population but not in another (e.g., as a result of treating cells with a stimulus that leads to the induction of certain genes). The colony or plaque lifts are first probed with labelled RNA from one population (say the noninduced cells). Once hybridizing colonies or plaques have been located, the labelled RNA is stripped from the membrane (usually by washing at a temperature greater than the melting temperature). The membrane is then probed with labelled RNA from the second population (in this case, the induced cells), and the hybridizing colonies or plaques are located. The colonies or plaques that hybridize in the second probing, but not in the first, correspond to sequences that are induced by whatever treatment was used. The approach can be made more sensitive by enriching the RNA from the second population (and also the library if necessary) for sequences that are absent from the first, as described in Section 4.4.6.

2. Chromosome walking. Successive rounds of screening of a genomic library with DNA probes can be used to assemble an ordered collection of clones located in a linear fashion down a chromosome. This procedure is often called *chromosome walking*. It is useful for obtaining sequences that are close on a chromosome to one for which a clone is already available, such as a nearby gene or restriction-fragment-length polymorphism marker. Starting with this clone, a genomic library is screened, and hybridizing clones are picked out. These will contain sequences overlapping with the first sequence to a greater or lesser extent. The degree of overlap can be assessed by Southern blotting and hybridization. Clones selected in this way are used to screen the genomic library again. Hybridizing clones are picked out, and their degree of overlap with the starting clone assessed. If there is little or no overlap, they must be further from the starting clone than those picked out in the first round of selection, as shown in Figure 5.5. The cycle is repeated, and each time, clones that are further from the original can be picked out. It may be possible to assess cytologically how far the clones have spread from the starting point by hybridization to chromosomes *in situ*.

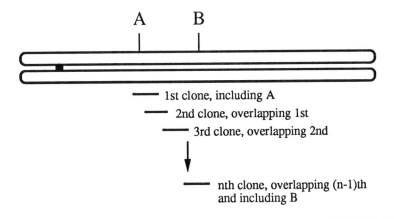

Figure 5.5 **Chromosome walking.** Starting from "A" on the chromosome, a series of overlapping clones is picked out by hybridization. Ultimately, "B" is reached.

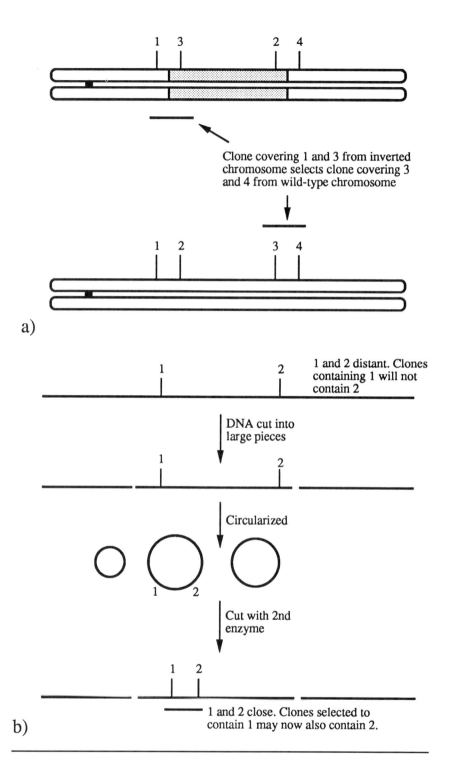

Figure 5.6 **Chromosome jumping.** In **(a)**, the aim is to jump from point 1 to point 4. In the upper chromosome, the intermediate region has been inverted. A clone covering 1 from the inverted chromosome includes material (covering 3) that is adjacent to it, but which is adjacent to 4 in the noninverted (lower) chromosome. The 1-3 clone can then be used to screen a library from the noninverted chromosome to pick out 3-4 clones. In **(b)**, regions of the genome are circularly permuted artificially by endonucle-ase digestion, circularization, and redigestion. That brings sequences that were initially far apart (1 and 2) close together.

With some organisms, it is be possible to use chromsomal inversions to "jump" along a chromosome rather than simply walk. Suppose we have a clone covering the endpoint of a region that is inverted in some strains. Probing a genomic library from a strain carrying the inversion allows you to select sequences from the other end of the inversion, as shown in Figure 5.6a. A different kind of jumping is shown in Figure 5.6b. Genomic DNA is cut into large pieces of 100–200 kb or so and circularized by intramolecular ligation. The circles are then cut with a second enzyme. This will open them out to generate molecules that have been permuted. A library is then made from these molecules, and clones hybridizing to the starting sequence are selected. However, these clones will also contain material that was originally as much as 100–200 kb away but which has been brought adjacent by the circularization-opening process.

3. **Breakpoint cloning.** This approach is used to identify the breakpoints of a reciprocal translocation, in which material has been exchanged between two chromosomes. These translocations are often identified as the cause of genetic disorders, and the ability to clone the sequences disrupted by the translocation may offer access to the genes that are affected. For example, translocations between the X chromosome and chromosome 21 have been implicated in a number of cases of Duchenne muscular dystrophy. Clones are selected from a library (made with one of the translocated chromosomes) that contain material hybridizing to the wild-type forms of both chromosomes involved in the rearrangement. These clones are likely to span the breakpoint itself (as shown in Figure 5.7).

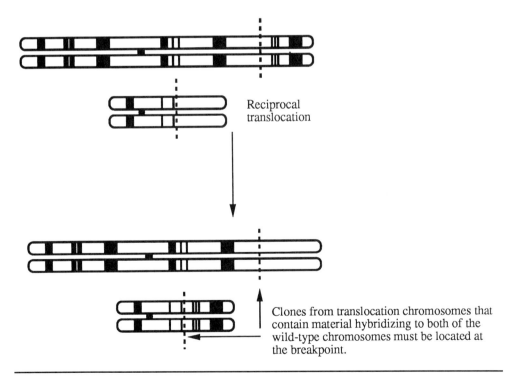

Reciprocal translocation

Clones from translocation chromosomes that contain material hybridizing to both of the wild-type chromosomes must be located at the breakpoint.

Figure 5.7 **Breakpoint cloning**. A reciprocal translocation has occurred between the upper two chromosomes to generate the lower ones. (Chromosome banding has been shown schematically to indicate this.)

4. Transposon tagging. This approach is applicable when the organism under study contains transposable genetic elements (often referred to as *transposons)* for which hybridization probes are available. These elements are DNA sequences that can move from one place in a chromosome to another, sometimes on the same chromosome and sometimes on a different one. This transposition may involve duplication of the element, with a copy left behind at the original site. Transposons are found in many bacterial, animal, and plant species. For transposon tagging to be feasible, it is not always necessary for transposons to occur naturally in the species in question. In some cases, they can be transferred from a species in which they do occur, into one in which they do not, by transformation, while retaining their ability to transpose.

Insertion of a transposable element into a gene often generates a recognizable mutant phenotype, such as an unstable inactivation of the gene. For transposon tagging, we need a strain carrying a mutation caused by such an insertion into the gene of interest. A genomic library is prepared from the mutant strain and screened with a probe for the transposable element. Clones that are picked out will contain the transposon and, flanking it, the gene of interest. If necessary, these clones can then be used to probe genomic libraries from wild-type organisms to obtain the intact gene.

Transposon tagging is complicated by the fact that there may be several copies of any given transposable element per genome, so it may not be possible to isolate the gene of interest unambiguously. Further screening of the clones selected may be necessary, using the other techniques outlined in this chapter. Sometimes a different strain has a mutation in the same gene, but caused by a different transposable element. This can be screened in exactly the same way, and the sequences that are picked out independently using both transposable elements are highly likely to be the ones of interest.

5. 2. 4 Expression of the coding function *in vitro*

There are three techniques for the expression of the coding function *in vitro*, although two rely on the hybridization of particular sequences (actually mRNA) to the libraries to be screened and therefore could also be regarded as belonging in the previous section. These methods require antibodies to the protein of interest and are all rather labour-intensive and costly and, therefore, best suited to the screening of smaller libraries. Although they could be used for screening cDNA libraries or libraries from very small genomes (such as organelles), they would not be suitable for screening eukaryotic nuclear genomic libraries.

1. Transcription and translation *in vitro*. In this technique, DNA constructs (usually plasmids) are isolated from the host and incubated in an extract capable of transcribing and translating them. This extract is often made from a lysate of *E. coli* cells and contains RNA polymerase, ribosomes, tRNAs, and so forth. Radiolabelled amino acids are used, so that any newly synthesized polypeptides can be readily detected. The products of the transcription-translation reactions are analysed by immunoprecipitation with antibodies to the protein in question, followed by electrophoresis of the immunoprecipitates in SDS-polyacrylamide gels and autoradiography or fluorography (as described in

Section 4.4.2). If a given construct is able to direct the synthesis of the relevant protein, the latter will be precipitated by the antibodies and subsequently detected in the gel.

When translation takes place concomitantly with transcription, the processes are said to be *coupled*. It is also possible to carry out the reactions separately, in *linked* reactions. Here the recombinants to be screened are incubated with a suitable RNA polymerase (which could be the *E. coli* enzyme or a more specialized one; see Section 1.3.2) to produce transcripts that are then translated in a separate reaction, normally by the use of a reticulocyte or wheat germ extract.

Transcription and translation *in vitro* relies on the ability of the extract to express the cloned sequences. Expression may well be possible for Gram-negative bacterial sequences (especially if the extract is from *E. coli*), but is much less likely for other sequences. Expression vectors may be helpful (see Section 8.2.2). The whole procedure from DNA isolation to SDS-polyacrylamide gel electrophoresis is very time-consuming. The effort can be reduced by screening the DNA constructs in pooled batches. Once a pooled batch has been identified as containing a suitable recombinant, the individual members (or smaller pools) can be screened.

2. Hybrid-released translation (HRT). This procedure is also called hybrid-selected translation, or HST. The approach uses hybridization to obtain RNA species that are complementary to individual DNA clones; we then translate the RNA *in vitro*, looking for clones that pick out the RNA coding for the protein of interest. The approach is shown in Figure 5.8. Cloned DNA is purified from the library, made single-stranded by alkali denaturation, and bound to a suitable solid-phase support, such as nitrocellulose. Different members of the library (A, B, and C in Figure 5.8) are bound to separate nitrocellulose filters and are then incubated with RNA from cells known to be making the protein of interest. (If we are screening a cDNA library, the RNA is often from the same preparation that was used to make the library.) After the filters are washed to remove nonspecifically bound RNA, the specifically bound material is eluted from each filter and translated separately *in vitro* in a reticulocyte lysate or wheat germ extract. Immunoprecipitation, SDS-polyacrylamide gel electrophoresis, and autoradiography are used to determine which translation reactions have led to the synthesis of the protein (and therefore which DNA species were able to hybridize to the RNA for that protein). As with transcription and translation, the approach is time-consuming, although again the effort can be reduced by screening pools of recombinants.

3. Hybrid-arrested translation (HART). This procedure resembles hybrid-released translation in some respects (see Figure 5.9). Samples of mRNA (known to include the mRNA for the protein of interest) are incubated with melted DNA constructs from individual recombinants (A, B, and C in Figure 5.9). After any annealing has taken place, the RNA is translated *in vitro* and the translation products are screened for the production of the desired protein. Because the annealing of DNA to RNA blocks translation of the RNA (possibly because the RNA:DNA hybrid molecules are particularly susceptible to nucleolytic attack in the translation extract), the clones of interest will be identifiable as those that specifically block the synthesis of the protein. As before, clones are generally screened in batches to reduce the effort involved.

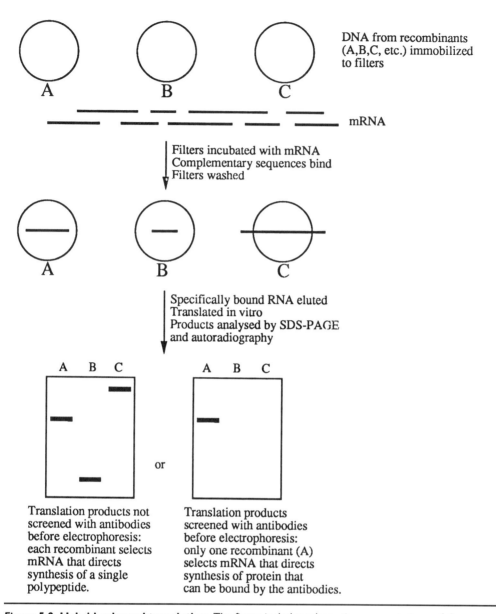

Figure 5.8 **Hybrid-released translation**. The figure includes schematic representations of the autoradiographs of SDS-gels that would be expected if translation products are electrophoresed without prior immunoprecipitation (lower left) and if translation products are screened with antibodies to the protein of interest and only the immunoprecipitated material is run in the gel (lower right).

5. 2. 5 How do I confirm that I've got the right clone?

Having isolated a cDNA or genomic clone, how do we confirm that it encodes a protein and, in particular, the protein that we are interested in? There are several features to look for:

1. ***Hpa*II tiny fragment islands.** In vertebrates, the presence of a gene in a piece of genomic DNA is often betrayed by the presence of large numbers of *Hpa*II

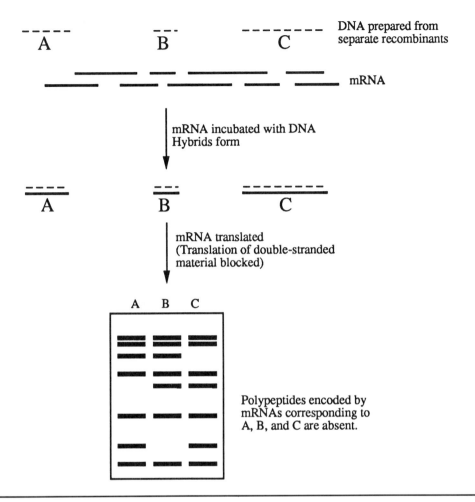

Figure 5.9 **Hybrid-arrested translation.**

sites. These generally mark the 5' end and are called *Hpa*II *tiny fragment islands*, because they give rise to tiny fragments on digestion with *Hpa*II. In fact, these regions are not really abnormally rich in *Hpa*II sites; it is more the case that other regions are deficient in them. This is because -CG- dinucleotides in these other regions tend to have the C methylated. However, the presence of 5-methylcytosine can be mutagenic, since it deaminates spontaneously to form thymine. There seems, therefore, to have been selection to reduce the number of -CG- dinucleotides in regions where methylation may occur, and this also has the effect of reducing the number of *Hpa*II sites (recognition sequence -CCGG-) in those regions. Methylation is less frequent in the vicinity of 5' ends of genes, so there is less selection against having -CG- dinucleotides in those regions, and hence there is a higher frequency of *Hpa*II sites. The presence of *Hpa*II tiny fragment islands in the genomic DNA we have isolated therefore suggests the presence of a gene.

2. Open reading frames. A common way of showing that a piece of DNA could encode a protein is to demonstrate the presence of an *open reading frame*, or ORF, in the nucleotide sequence. An ORF comprises an initiation codon followed by a long stretch without any termination codons in the same reading frame (unless the protein encoded is very small). However, if the gene contains introns, these will interrupt the ORF and may make it difficult to detect. This will not be a problem with cDNA.

3. Nonrandom base composition. The requirement to encode an amino acid sequence imposes a nonrandom distribution of bases on the DNA, which can be detected by computer analysis. Because introns do not usually have a coding function, it may be possible to distinguish them from exons, as the former will have a more random base composition.

4. Nature of the gene product. If you have found an open reading frame, you can use the genetic code to predict the amino acid sequence of the product and compare it with the protein of interest or with proteins of related function. If you know the biological activity of the protein (if it is an enzyme, for example), you may be able to assay for it in cells containing the cloned DNA.

5. Distribution. If you have neither an amino acid sequence for comparisons, nor an assay, things are more difficult. You can use Northern analysis to check that the tissue or developmental distribution of mRNA from the gene you have cloned agrees with the distribution of the protein you are interested in. At the protein level, you may be able to generate antibodies to the protein that is encoded in your clone and use them to look at that protein's distribution. If it is the same as the distribution of the protein you are interested in, it is further evidence that you have the right clone.

6. Mutations. Using the techniques described in Section 7.7, you can generate organisms with mutations in the gene you have cloned. If these also lack the protein you are interested in, it again suggests you have the right clone.

5. 2. 6 Choosing a strategy

For a probability "P" of having a particular sequence in a collection of recombinants, each of which has an insert equivalent to a fraction "x" of the genome, the collection must have $\ln(1 - P)/\ln(1 - x)$ recombinants. Therefore, to have a 99% chance of finding a sequence in a library of, say, 20-kb fragments cloned from a genome of 3×10^6 kb, about 700,000 recombinants would have to be screened. This is rather a lot to handle easily; it corresponds to a total amount of DNA over four times larger than the genome and assumes that the screening process is fully reliable and that all copies of the sequence will be detected. Even for a 75% chance, over 200,000 recombinants would have to be screened, which is still a lot of recombinants. A cDNA library, however, is enriched for those sequences that are actually expressed, so a smaller number of recombinants need to be screened to obtain the sequence corresponding to a given protein. If the cDNA library was constructed using a tissue in which mRNA for the protein was particularly abundant, the number of recombinants to be screened could be reduced still further. This would also be the case using one of the specialized libraries described in Section 4.4.

    Exactly how a particular library is to be screened will depend on a number of factors. These include the size of the library, the vector in which the library is constructed, and the availability of antibodies, amino acid sequence, hybridization probes, and mutants. There are no hard and fast rules for screening; the following are intended as guidelines for obtaining three types of genes.

1.   Genes from small genomes (e.g., viruses and organelles). When genes are to be obtained from small genomes, the number of recombinants to be screened will be small, so labour-intensive methods – such as expression *in vitro* and even DNA sequencing of clones – may be acceptable. If mutant complementation is possible, use that. If long DNA hybridization probes are available, use those. If not, use oligonucleotide probes based on amino acid sequence, immunochemical screening, or expression *in vitro* (if antibodies are available).

2.   Bacterial genes. To obtain bacterial genes, screen genomic libraries. It is rarely necessary to bother with cDNA libraries, which may be difficult to make anyway, because of the lack of polyA tails on mRNA. If mutant complementation is possible, use that. If not, use hybridization probes if available, or else immunochemical screening or oligonucleotide probing, depending on the availability of antibodies or amino acid sequence. As a last resort, use expression *in vitro*.

3.   Eukaryotic genes. In some circumstances, mutant complementation may be a possible way to obtain eukaryotic genes. If available, use hybridization probes on genomic or cDNA libraries. If not, use immunochemical screening or oligonucleotide probing of cDNA libraries according to the availability of antibodies or amino acid sequence. Then use cDNA clones to probe genomic libraries, if necessary. As a last resort, use hybrid-released or hybrid-arrested translation.

Eukaryotes vary widely in the sizes of their genomes, and it may be easier to find the gene first in a "model" organism with a small genome. You can then use that as a probe to find the gene in a larger genome if you need to. For example, *Arabidopsis* is often used as a model plant. In comparison with many plants, it has a very small haploid genome of about 70,000 kb. Maize, by contrast, has a haploid genome of about 3×10^6 kb. With *Arabidopsis,* you would need to screen 16,000 genomic clones with 20-kb inserts to have a 99% chance of finding a particular sequence, rather than the 700,000 that would need to be screened with maize. *Arabidopsis* has other advantages over many other plants – in particular, its small size and short generation time.

5. 3   SCREENING FOR OTHER FUNCTIONS: REPORTER GENES

5. 3. 1   Promoters

A number of vectors exist for identifying sequences that are able to function as promoters *in vivo*. They are usually called promoter-probe vectors, and Figure 5.10 shows a typical example. It contains a gene called the reporter gene (in this case, for chloramphenicol acetyltransferase), from which the promoter has been removed, preceded by a multiple cloning site. DNA is inserted into this cloning site, and recombinants are introduced into a suitable host. After selection for plasmid uptake (in this case, by ampicillin resistance), transformants can be selected for chloramphenicol resistance. These transformants should have acquired a promoter in the cloning site directing transcription of the chloramphenicol resistance gene. Alternatively, chloramphenicol acetyltransferase

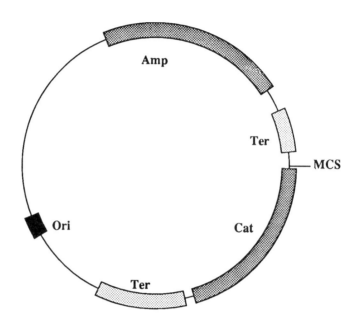

Figure 5.10 Promoter-probe vector pKK232-8 (5.1 kb). The promoterless reporter gene (Cat) is for chloramphenicol acetyltransferase. Sequences for promoter screening are inserted into the multiple cloning site MCS. Ter sequences are transcription terminators. Amp is the gene for ampicillin resistance, and Ori is the origin of replication.

activity can be assayed to get a quantitative measure of promoter activity. Note that the promoter-probe region is flanked in this vector by terminators (from the *E. coli rrnB* operon), because very powerful promoters in the cloning site might interfere with other aspects of plasmid function, such as the ampicillin resistance. Other indicators of promoter activity besides antibiotic resistance can be used. These include

a. nutritional markers, such as *gal*K for galactokinase (allowing growth on galactose as a sole carbon source for a cell which is otherwise *galK⁻*), and

b. the genes for luciferase, beta-galactosidase, and beta-glucuronidase. Activity of the latter two can be detected using the chromogenic substrates X-Gal (see Section 2.3.2) and its glucuronide equivalent, X-Gluc (see Section 9.6.6).

Caution should be used when interpreting the results of experiments using promoter probes. The characteristics of promoters vary widely from species to species (both in sequence and in the proteins that bind to them), and it is quite possible that a sequence that is a promoter in one organism will not function as a promoter in *E. coli* and *vice versa*. The more closely related the source of the insert DNA to *E. coli*, the more reliable promoter-probe vectors will be. There is no certainty of reliability even with *E. coli* DNA, as many promoters require a control signal (perhaps a nutrient in the medium) for activation. If this control signal is not supplied when the screening is carried out, promoters responsive to it are unlikely to be detected.

Promoter-probe vectors for many organisms besides *E. coli* are available. They all work on the same principle of assaying for the expression of a promoterless gene from a piece of inserted DNA. A similar approach is often used to determine the effects of sequence modification on known promoters that have already been cloned. The modified promoters are introduced into the host organism and the activity of the reporter gene monitored.

5. 3. 2 Transcription terminators

Terminator-probe vectors work on a principle similar to that of promoter-probe vectors. Putative terminators are inserted between a promoter and a reporter gene. Terminator function can then be assayed by measuring the reduction in reporter gene expression. Direct selection for terminator function is also possible. Figure 5.11 shows an example using the *galK* gene (for galactokinase). Expression of this gene in a cell that is mutant for *galT*, which encodes galactose-1-phosphate uridylyl transferase (the next step in galactose metabolism), is lethal because of the buildup of galactose-1-phosphate. So the terminator-probe vector is used in a *galK⁻galT⁻* host. If there is no terminator between the promoter and the plasmid *galK*, the cell is phenotypically *galT⁻* and is killed by galactose. If there is a terminator, the cell will be *galK⁻galT⁻* and therefore resistant to galactose. This allows the selection of sequences that have terminator activity in *E. coli*, but only under the conditions of growth on an agar plate. That does not necessarily give a conclusive indication of terminator activity under different conditions or in a different organism.

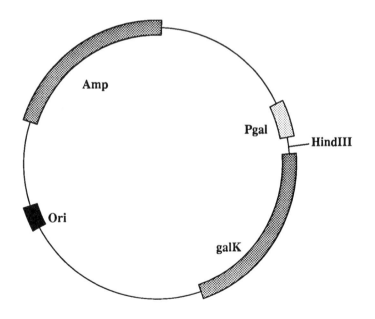

Figure 5.11 **Terminator-probe vector pKG1800 (4.9 kb).** Pgal is a promoter for *galK*, expression of which is lethal in a *galT⁻* background in the presence of galactose. Amp is the gene for ampicillin resistance, and Ori is the origin of replication.

5. 3. 3 Autonomously replicating sequences

It is also possible to select for sequences that can function as origins of replication. These are sometimes called *autonomously replicating sequences,* or ARS elements. The first step in selecting for ARS is to remove the physiological origin of replication from a plasmid by digestion with a suitable restriction enzyme. The DNA under study is then ligated in its place, and the recombinants are introduced into *E. coli*. Selection is then imposed for a selectable marker on the plasmid. The removal of the plasmid's origin of replication means that stable propagation in the host is no longer possible and that the marker cannot be retained. If a particular DNA sequence inserted into the plasmid contains a sequence able to act as an origin of replication, stable propagation of the plasmid is possible, and the marker can be selected and retained. The same problems of interpretation of the results apply as with promoter- and terminator-probe vectors. A further problem is that in some cases the probe plasmid may integrate (by legitimate or illegitimate recombination) into the host chromosome during the course of selection. It will therefore be stably propagated as part of the host chromosome, even though it does not necessarily have its own ARS element, and will give rise to colonies in the selection procedure. The likelihood that this will occur can be greatly reduced by the use of a recombination-deficient host.

CHAPTER

6

Polymerase
Chain Reaction

6. 1 THE BASIC TECHNIQUE

6. 1. 1 The method

The techniques described so far for the amplification of specific DNA sequences can often be replaced by a direct enzymatic amplification process called the *polymerase chain reaction*, or PCR for short. The basic procedure is outlined in Figure 6.1. In the simplest case, PCR amplification requires that we know a small amount of nucleotide sequence at each end of the region to be amplified. Oligonucleotides complementary to those sequences are synthesized, typically 20 or so nucleotides long. These oligonucleotides are used as primers for enzymatic amplification.

A reaction mixture is first set up containing the sample of DNA for amplification, the primers in large molar excess, dNTPs, and a heat-stable DNA polymerase. The most common enzyme for this purpose is the *Taq* polymerase – DNA polymerase isolated from the thermophilic bacterium *Thermus aquaticus*, which can be grown routinely in the lab at 75°C or higher. This enzyme, which the bacterium uses for cellular DNA synthesis, has a temperature optimum of at least 80°C and is not denatured by the repeated heating and cooling cycles that we shall see are needed in the amplification process. There are many other thermophilic bacteria, and their polymerases can also be used.

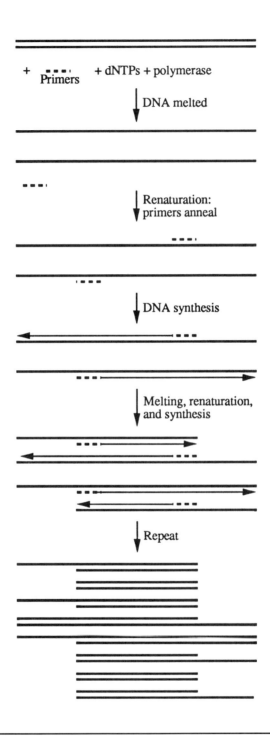

Figure 6.1 **Polymerase chain reaction.**

The mixture is heated to a temperature sufficient to melt (i.e., separate the strands of) the sample DNA. After this, it is cooled to a temperature low enough for the primers to anneal to it. Of course, it is possible for the sample DNA simply to self-anneal, but this is rendered less likely by the large molar excess of the primers. The mix is then incubated at a temperature sufficient for the polymerase to synthesize a complementary strand to each piece of sample DNA, starting with the primers and using the dNTPs provided. We have therefore doubled the number of copies of the target region we are interested in. After this round of DNA synthesis, the mixture is heated for strand separation again, cooled again for primer annealing, and incubated for another round of DNA synthesis. Each time the cycle is carried out, there is a doubling of the number of copies of the target region between the primer annealing sites. A typical set of reactions might have an initial melting carried out for 5 minutes at 92°C, followed by 30 cycles each comprising melting for 1 minute at 92°C, renaturation for 1 minute at 60°C, and DNA synthesis for 1.5 minutes at 72°C, and then after the 30 cycles, a final extended round of DNA synthesis for 10 minutes. This would result in a theoretical amplification of over 10^9-fold. Applied even to a single DNA molecule of 1 kb, that would generate 1 ng of DNA, just about sufficient to see in a gel by staining with ethidium bromide.

Because of the repetitive nature of the process, it lends itself to automation, and many companies market *thermal cyclers* or *PCR machines*, which will carry out a series of programmed cycles of heating and cooling. Because the polymerase is thermostable and the primers were added in large excess initially, there is no need for further additions during the reaction – temperature control is all that is required.

Notice that not all the molecules generated will be of defined length. If this process is applied to genomic DNA (call this "full-length" material), half the molecules will be full-length after the first cycle, and the other half will start with a primer and have an undefined end, determined by how far the polymerase progressed during DNA synthesis (call these "half-length" molecules). In the next cycle, each full-length molecule will generate one full-length and one half-length molecule, and each half-length molecule will generate one half-length one and one fully defined target molecule (beginning and ending at the primer sites), as shown in Figure 6.1. As each cycle proceeds, the number of full-length molecules remains constant, the number of half-length molecules increases arithmetically, and the number of target molecules increases essentially geometrically. After many cycles, gel electrophoresis of PCR products will therefore indicate, to all intents and purposes, molecules all of a single size, corresponding to a single band in the gel.

If the sequences flanking the target region are not known precisely, it may still be possible to use PCR, with mixed oligonucleotide primers or primers that contain modified bases, such as inosine. These primers are analogous to the mixed or inosine-containing oligonucleotides that are sometimes used as hybridization probes (Section 5.2.3). So, for example, it might be possible to amplify sequences encoding different members of a gene family using a single set of primers corresponding to highly (but not necessarily totally) conserved regions of the gene.

6. 1. 2 Applications

Because PCR is automated and a typical set of cycles can be carried out simultaneously on many separate samples in a few hours, and starting amounts of

DNA can be vanishingly small, PCR has a number of applications where standard cloning techniques might be inappropriate – for example, where speed or the number of samples to be processed is important, or when the amount of DNA available is very limited. Here are some of the applications:

1. Diagnostic. PCR is useful as a diagnostic tool – for example, in the identification of specific genetic traits and for the detection of pathogens. One of the first applications of PCR to genetic diagnosis was for sickle cell anaemia, allowing analysis to be completed within a day rather than the weeks taken by the conventional approach of hybridization analysis of DNA from cells. The sickle cell mutation in the beta globin gene destroys a restriction site, and the test involved PCR amplification of this region of the genome and analysis of the PCR products for the presence or absence of the restriction site. In general, PCR products can be analysed by

a. use of restriction enzymes, although it is rare for a mutation to create or destroy a restriction site,

b. determining whether an oligonucleotide probe specific for a particular allele is able to hybridize to PCR products, or

c. sequencing the PCR products directly (see Section 6.2.4).

Tests for the presence of particular pathogens can be made using primers specific for the genomes of those organisms. This permits detection at extremely low levels.

2. Forensic. The ability to amplify DNA from regions of the genome that are highly polymorphic (and are therefore variable between individuals) starting with samples containing very small amounts of DNA (for example, single hairs, or traces of body fluids such as blood and semen), leads to applications in forensic work. A number of polymorphic regions have been used as targets for amplification, including the D loop of mitochondrial DNA (mitochondrial DNA also has the advantage of being present at a high copy number per cell), which is highly variable between individuals (much more so than the rest of the mitochondrial genome); the tandemly repeated *minisatellites* used in conventional genetic fingerprinting; and human leucocyte antigen (HLA) sequences. In a celebrated case reported in 1991, the technique was applied to the skeletal remains of a murder victim who had been wrapped in a carpet and buried from 1981 until the discovery of the bones in 1989. DNA isolated from these bones was heavily degraded, to fragments of less than 300 nucleotides, so analysis by conventional genetic fingerprinting techniques involving restriction digestion, Southern blotting, and hybridization would not have been possible. The poor condition of the DNA also made PCR amplification of minisatellites impracticable, so amplification of shorter *microsatellite* regions, composed of varying numbers of copies of the simple repeated sequence -CA-, was used. PCR products from the victim were matched with those from the putative mother and father, and the provisional identification of the body, which had been made earlier on the basis of facial reconstruction and dental records, was confirmed.

3. Archaeology, palaeontology, and evolution. The age of tissue that can be subjected to PCR is certainly not limited to a few years, and it is often possible to amplify DNA from ancient museum specimens and archaeological remains. Multiple copy sequences, such as mitochondrial DNA or chloroplast DNA, are a particularly useful target. Comparison of polymorphic sequences from the ancient DNA with sequences observed today allows inferences to be made about the origins of particular populations or species. For example, the thylacine or marsupial wolf has been extinct for some time, although it was once a wide-spread species in Australia. Morphological data led to controversy over whether it was more closely related in evolution to a group of South American marsupial carnivores or to other Australian species such as the Tasmanian devil. Mitochondrial DNA was successfully amplified by PCR from skin and museum specimens collected in the late 19th and early 20th centuries. The sequence of the amplified DNA was determined, and it was interpreted as showing that the thylacine was more closely related to the Australian species than to the South American ones, and that the morphological similarities to the South American ones resulted from convergent evolution.

If the method of preservation was suitable, DNA can be isolated from very old samples indeed, such as 20-million-year-old insect remains preserved in amber. However, even though material may be heavily degraded, it may be possible to amplify larger sequences as a result of *jumping PCR*, described in Section 6.3.5.

4. Present-day population genetics. The ability to amplify material rapidly from a large number of DNA preparations leads to applications in population genetics, such as the determination of frequencies of particular alleles in a large collection of individuals. Using specific primers, it may be possible to amplify DNA from an organism that cannot be separated from organisms of another species, such as bacteria that cannot be cultured axenically.

6. 2 MODIFICATIONS

6. 2. 1 Hard copies

Having amplified a specific DNA fragment, we may find it convenient to insert a copy of the products into a vector for subsequent cloning and maintenance by conventional means; this is often called "making a hard copy". This can be achieved by blunt-end ligation of PCR products into the vector or by digestion of the amplified molecules with a restriction enzyme if suitable sites are present at, or close to, their ends. If there are no suitable sites present, they can be added by inclusion at the ends of the primers before amplification, as shown in Figure 6.2. The primers will anneal to the target DNA, with the restriction site sequences unbound. The half-length molecules that are formed will have the restriction site present at one end, and all the target-length DNA molecules will have the sites at both ends. The amplified molecules can then be cut at their ends with the appropriate enzyme(s) and the fragments cloned in the usual way. When designing primers for this purpose, it is usual to include a few nucleotides of nonspecific sequence beyond the restriction site, because sites at the very ends of molecules may not be cut efficiently. It may be necessary to avoid using particular enzymes to cut within those primer sequences if they also have sites within the target region.

6. 2. 2 Inverse PCR

The result of the standard approach outlined so far is the amplification of sequence between the primer annealing sites. However, it is also possible to

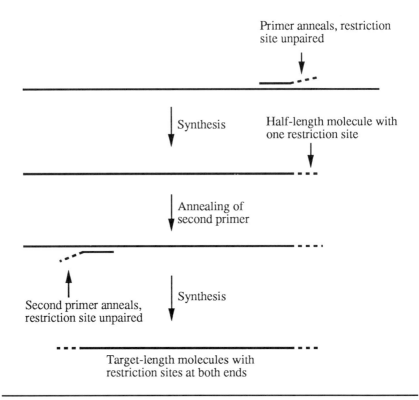

Figure 6.2 **Addition of restriction sites in PCR.** The dashed region indicates a part of the primer that contains a restriction site not present in the target DNA.

arrange for the amplification of sequences *outside* the primers, in a technique called *inverse polymerase chain reaction,* or IPCR. The approach is summarized in Figure 6.3. The sample DNA is first cut with an enzyme outside the region whose sequence is already known. The resulting linear molecules are then circularized by ligation, under conditions that favour intramolecular reactions rather than intermolecular ones. A second restriction digestion is then done, using an enzyme cutting *within* the region of known sequence. The result is that the first fragment containing this sequence has been "turned inside out", leaving known sequence on the outside and the material that had previously been flanking it, within. Primers complementary to the known sequence on the outside of the molecule can now be used to amplify the region of interest between them.

The IPCR technique is especially powerful when combined with transposon tagging (see Section 5.2.3). If a previously characterized transposon inserts into a gene of interest (detected by alteration of its expression – usually unstably inactivating it – and resulting in an identifiable phenotype), then the gene can be amplified using IPCR and primers from the transposon sequence.

6. 2. 3 Mutagenesis

Perfect matching between the primer and the target DNA is not necessary, provided allowance is made for this in determining the conditions for primer annealing. The technique can therefore be used to engineer specific mutations in the amplified sequence by constructing a primer that corresponds to the mutated sequence, rather than to the original.

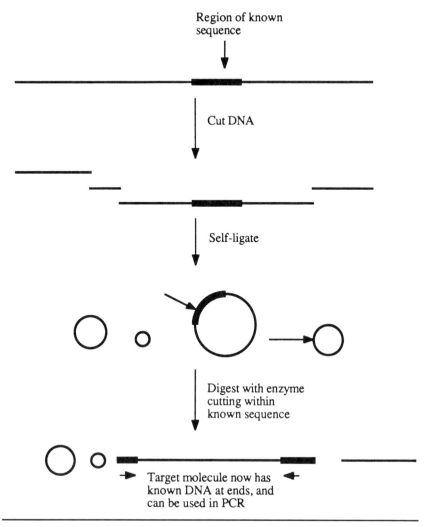

Figure 6.3 Inverse PCR (IPCR).

6. 2. 4   Sequencing ,

By reducing the amount of one of the two primers, it is possible to arrange for preferential amplification of one of the strands, resulting in a preparation of effectively single-stranded DNA, which can then be used directly for sequencing. The other amplification primer can then also serve as a primer for the sequencing reactions. (Of course, it would also be possible to clone the amplification products into a vector suitable for sequencing, such as M13.) Preferential amplification of one strand in this way is known as *asymmetric PCR*. Single-stranded material can also be obtained by tagging one of the primers (with biotin, for example) and then using an affinity purification method (streptavidin-based, if biotin was used) to separate the tagged strand.

6. 2. 5   Anchored PCR

Anchored PCR is applied when only one piece of sequence (and therefore one priming site) for the region of interest is known. The aim is to attach the region

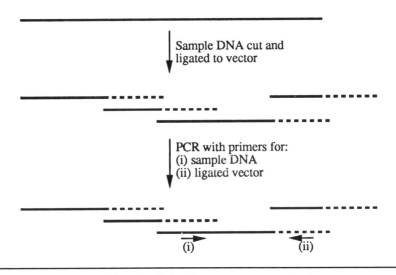

Figure 6.4 **Anchored PCR.** The dashed line represents a molecule of known sequence that provides one of the two priming sites for PCR. The primers are shown by (i) and (ii).

to be amplified to a piece of known sequence and then use that to act as the second priming site. There are two ways in which this can most easily be done. In one (Figure 6.4) the *anchor* sequence for the second priming site is added by ligation – for example, into a vector. The target DNA is first cut with a suitable enzyme and the fragments are ligated into a vector of known sequence. (If this is a standard vector molecule, we are in effect using a library.) Amplification is then carried out with two primers, one of which is to the region of known sequence and the other to the vector sequence directly flanking the site of target DNA insertion. In the second approach, the sample DNA is again fragmented before the first synthesis, which uses the primer for the known region. After synthesis with that primer, the resulting DNA fragments are tailed with a run of, say, G residues added by terminal deoxynucleotidyl transferase and dGTP. Oligo-dC can then be annealed to the oligo-dG tail and used to prime the second synthesis. (If the target molecule is a piece of polyA$^+$ RNA, then – depending on where the known sequence lies – it may be possible to use the polyA tail as a first priming site and the short stretch of known sequence as the second. The first synthesis reaction, on the mRNA template, would of course use reverse transcriptase, rather than *Taq* DNA polymerase.)

6. 3   PRECAUTIONS AND DRAWBACKS

6. 3. 1   Size

A number of factors impose a size limit on the fragments that can be amplified. In practice, this limit seems to be a few kilobases.

6. 3. 2   Amplifying the wrong sequence

PCR depends on the availability of a certain amount of sequence information and the ability of the primers to anneal to the correct sequence. The latter depends on the conditions used (ionic concentration, temperature, etc.) as well

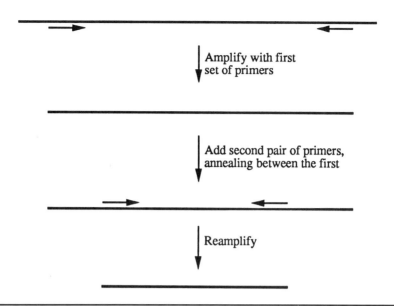

Figure 6.5 **PCR with nested primers.**

as the actual sequence of the primers. It is possible for primers to anneal to the "wrong" part of the target DNA through chance complementarity. If this happens and the primers are also in the correct orientation to each other (i.e., directing synthesis towards each other) and at sites that are not too far apart, the result is the amplification of a sequence other than the desired one. That result might be detectable if the size of the amplification products (as estimated by gel electrophoresis) is different from that expected – but prior knowledge of the size is not always available. The possibility of incorrect annealing may be avoided by use of longer primers, which will be more specific.

Use of sets of *nested* primers may also help to avoid the amplification of the wrong region. Amplification is carried out first using one pair of primers, and the products of this amplification are further amplified using another pair of primers, which anneal within the amplified region (Figure 6.5). Incorrect amplification would therefore require *both* pairs of primers to anneal incorrectly, with the second pair able to do so within the amplified sequence, which is unlikely.

If a primer contains internal secondary structure, it may self-anneal, forming a hairpin. This is likely to prevent the primer's annealing to the sample DNA and, therefore, to prevent amplification. The potential to form secondary structure should therefore be avoided when the primers are designed.

6. 3. 3   Contamination

Because of the extraordinary sensitivity of PCR, there is a particular danger of contamination by extraneous material of the DNA sample to be amplified. This might be of laboratory origin (for example, from aerosols created by the pipetting of solutions containing related DNA sequences) or of external origin (perhaps by bacterial, fungal, or human contamination of sample tissue).

Laboratory contamination (for example, with DNA carried as aerosols) can be minimized by precautions such as careful use and design of pipettes, and separation of the pre-PCR and post-PCR stages of an experiment into different rooms. Contamination from other sources can be reduced by careful handling and preparation of a sample before amplification (e.g., by avoiding direct contact with human skin, and by removal of surface layers of the sample before DNA extraction, as these may be more heavily contaminated). Careful selection of primers may also help; for example, if obtaining mitochondrial DNA from human bones, the use of human-specific primers reduces the chance that contaminating fungal mitochondrial DNA will be amplified. Use of appropriate negative controls is also important, such as carrying out PCR using material from a "dummy" DNA extraction with no sample tissue added, to indicate the presence of any PCR-amplifiable contamination in buffers or in other reagents, or as aerosols. It is often the case that DNA from archaeological specimens is degraded, so that only short sequences of a few hundred base pairs or less can be amplified. Amplification of long sequences from archaeological specimens may be indicative of contamination with recent DNA. (This is not always the case, though; see "Jumping PCR," Section 6.3.5.)

6. 3. 4 Sequence heterogeneity

Amplification may give rise to a mixture of molecules of slightly differing sequences. A mixture could arise for several reasons.

1. Heterozygosity. If the sample DNA came from an individual heterozygous at the locus in question, each of the alleles present should be represented in similar quantities in the PCR products. This can easily be detected by direct sequencing of the PCR products (see Section 6.2.4), since it gives rise to two bands at the same level – but in different tracks – in the sequencing gel. However, if products are cloned before the sequencing, the heterogeneity will not be detected if only a single recombinant is used for sequencing (as individual recombinants are derived from single PCR product molecules). Indeed, the heterogeneity may – by chance – go undetected even if several recombinants are used.

2. Population heterogeneity. If the DNA came not from a single individual, but from several, then heterogeneity in the population will give rise to heterogeneity in the products. In this case, there may be many different alleles to identify.

3. DNA damage and polymerase error. Heterogeneity can also arise from damage to DNA before amplification, especially if the sample has not been carefully preserved. This is therefore particularly likely to be a problem with archaeological and forensic material. Damage includes oxidation or deamination of bases and chemical crosslinking (within or between strands). As well as slowing down the polymerase (possibly resulting in the preferential amplification of undamaged – and perhaps contaminating – DNA), these changes may lead to the incorporation of incorrect bases during amplification. If direct sequencing of amplified products is carried out, this misincorporation may not be a problem, because the sample molecule that caused the misincorporation will be only a small proportion of the total number (unless the number of sample molecules is exceptionally small or the *same* site has been affected in all the sample molecules). Therefore, the erroneous sequence will have a weaker signal in the sequencing gel than does the genuine one. However, sequencing of a cloned PCR product might lead to the generation of an erroneous sequence, as the cloned product derives from a single molecule and the sequencing gel will show only one sequence.

The polymerase may also make spontaneous errors not resulting from damage to the sample DNA. The purified *Taq* polymerase lacks a 3'–5' exonuclease proofreading activity, giving an error rate of about 1 in 10,000 base pairs. Although this may seem rather low, after many cycles of PCR it would be more significant, and is likely to present a problem if sequencing is carried out on cloned individual PCR products.

Errors introduced by the polymerase, whether or not they result from template damage, can be expected to be evenly distributed over all three codon positions, whereas sequence heterogeneity (in coding regions) resulting from genuine allelic differences is likely to be concentrated in the third codon position and will have a tendency not to lead to amino acid substitutions.

6. 3. 5 Jumping PCR

When degraded DNA is amplified, it may be that any given sample molecule is not long enough to span the entire distance between the two priming sites. The result in the first round of synthesis would be extension of the primer to the end of a fragmented molecule, but not all the way to the second primer site. However, on a subsequent round of synthesis, the truncated amplification product may anneal to a different DNA fragment, which contains the remaining region intact (see Figure 6.6). This would then allow synthesis of the full

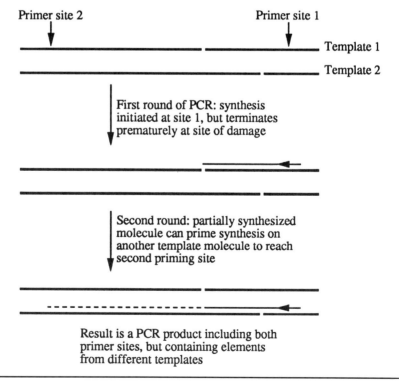

Figure 6.6 Jumping PCR. Although neither template molecule spans the entire distance between the priming sites, chimaeric molecules spanning this distance can be generated by template switching in successive rounds.

PCR product	1	ACCGATTAGCTTAATATATGCATGGATTAGTTCCAGGTATTTA
	2	G
	3	G C
	4	G C
	5	G C
	6	
	7	
	8	
	9	G C
	10	
	11	G C
	12	G

Figure 6.7 **Interpretation of PCR.** The figure shows the result of sequencing 12 cloned PCR products. Only the differences between products 2–12 and product 1 are marked. Products 1, 6, 7, 8, and 10 are identical (Type A). Products 3, 4, 5, 9, and 11 are identical (Type B), differing from Type A at two sites and probably representing a different allele. Product 2 is unique and may represent damaged DNA or a rare allele. Product 12 is also unique, but a hybrid between Types A and B. It could represent damaged DNA, another rare allele, or jumping PCR between Type A and Type B molecules.

PCR product. So it is sometimes possible to generate PCR products that are longer that any individual template molecule, which can be highly advantageous when amplifying badly degraded DNA. On the other hand, jumping PCR has the distinct disadvantage of creating chimaeric sequences that were not present initially. For example, if an individual is heterozygous at two sites within an amplified region, jumping PCR can generate molecules recombinant for these loci.

6. 3. 6 Interpretation

Interpreting the results of the sequencing of PCR products from potentially damaged DNA (especially if it may have come from a mixture of individuals) necessitates answering the following questions:

1. Which nucleotides occur infrequently at a heterogeneous site? (The rare nucleotides may be the results of damage to the template.)

2. If, at a number of sites within the molecule, there are apparently genuine allelic differences (i.e., similar numbers of each nucleotide at a heterogeneous site):

   a. Which *combinations* of sequences occur frequently (and are probably genuine alleles)?

   b. Which occur rarely (and might therefore be results of jumping PCR)?

A theoretical example is given in Figure 6.7.

CHAPTER

7

Modification and Mutagenesis

7.1 INTRODUCTION

So far, we have seen how to clone particular sequences and identify them. In Chapter 8 we will look at how these clones can be put to use directly at the DNA level and also to direct the synthesis of RNA and protein. However, it is often the case that we need to modify sequences before using them. Here are just three of the many situations in which we may need to do this:

a. We are trying to identify promoters and need to make a mutation in a putative promoter sequence to see if that actually affects the efficiency of transcription initiation.

b. We are interested in how the primary and higher order structures of a protein determine its function. It might therefore be necessary to modify the codon for a residue we believe to be at the active site of an enzyme and then assess the effects of that change on catalytic activity. Directed alteration of particular parts of proteins as a way of probing the relationship between structure and function or of altering the function in a controlled way is termed *protein engineering*, and the ability to make such changes through the DNA has resulted in a huge expansion of work in this area.

c. Genes are often cloned without our knowing the role that the proteins they encode have in the cell. Assessing that role may be possible by inactivating the endogenous gene in an organism to generate a mutant strain. This approach is often called *reverse genetics*, to emphasize the contrast with the more conventional approach whereby a strain carrying a mutation with specific effects is characterized first, and the relevant gene cloned and analysed subsequently.

Just what kind of mutation is needed – deletion, insertion, substitution, and so on – will depend upon the particular biological problem being pursued. The kind of mutation that is feasible depends upon the characteristics of the sequence involved – in particular, upon the distribution of restriction sites. Having constructed a mutation, it is very important to verify by appropriate techniques (restriction mapping, DNA sequencing, etc.) that the right mutation has indeed been made and also that no others have been created unintentionally as a result of the techniques used. The approaches taken can be divided broadly into two classes: those that rely on oligonucleotide-directed enzymatic synthesis of DNA, and those that do not. We will deal with the latter category first.

7. 2 ALTERATION OF RESTRICTION SITES

7. 2. 1 Removal

Sites can be removed by the procedure outlined in Figure 7.1. DNA is cut with the restriction enzyme whose site we wish to remove, to leave staggered ends. These are then rendered flush either by filling in with DNA polymerase or by degradation with a suitable exonuclease, as described in Section 1.3. The ends are then religated. The net result is a small insertion or deletion that destroys the recognition site. Re-treatment with the restriction enzyme will linearize any molecules in which the site was not successfully disrupted. A number of problems may be encountered in this approach.

1. There may be multiple restriction sites. There may be several target sites for the enzyme in the molecule. In this case, the initial digestion should be a partial one, so that molecules are on average cut at only one site. It is necessary to map the molecules generated to find one with the right site(s) destroyed.

2. The enzyme does not give staggered ends. In this case, it is necessary to engineer a small deletion at the site using exonuclease (see Section 1.3.3) or a small insertion (see Section 7.3.1).

3. We may disrupt a functional sequence. If the restriction site occurs in a functional sequence, such as a promoter or a protein-coding region, removal of the site may have undesirable consequences. This is particularly likely to be true if protein-coding regions are concerned, since the procedure outlined in Figure 7.1 normally generates insertions or deletions of 2 or 4 base pairs (because most sticky ends are of 2 or 4 bases); the procedure will therefore introduce a frameshift mutation into an open reading frame (since the sequence will be read in triplets). It may be possible to avoid this problem by introducing a slightly larger insertion or deletion.

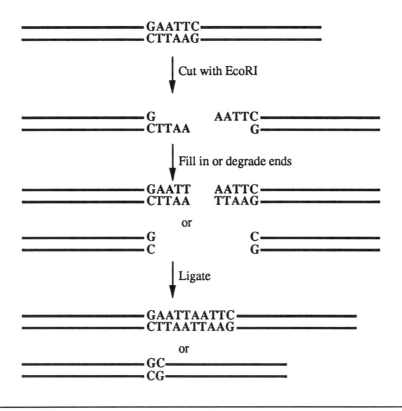

Figure 7.1 **Deletion of a restriction site.**

7. 2. 2 Creation

Creation of additional restriction sites at an existing restriction site can be done by the insertion of a suitable oligonucleotide, usually chemically synthesized, carrying the appropriate sequence(s). An important example of this is the construction of the polylinker sequence in the pUC and M13 vectors. This was achieved initially by insertion of the polylinker oligonucleotide into an *Eco*RI site in the *lacZ* minigene.

7. 3 INSERTIONS AND DELETIONS

7. 3. 1 Insertions

Insertions are quite easily constructed, usually by cutting at a suitable restriction site and then filling in the sticky ends with DNA polymerase, or by ligating in a chemically synthesized oligonucleotide or a suitable restriction fragment from elsewhere.

7. 3. 2 Deletions

Small deletions at a restriction site can be constructed by cutting and degrading the single-stranded ends with an exonuclease. Alternatively, a complete restriction fragment can be excised and the molecule religated. Sets of unidirectional or bidirectional deletions can be generated as described in Section 1.3.3. Sometimes a series of deleted regions (for example, in a putative promoter) is replaced by some other DNA fragment of equal length so as not to disrupt the spacing between other control regions. This is called *linker scanning*.

7. 4   POINT MUTATIONS: EARLY METHODS

The methods described so far bring about the insertion or deletion of several bases at a time. It is often necessary to alter a single base; that is, to bring about a *point mutation*. The early techniques have generally been superseded by oligonucleotide-directed mutagenesis, but it is worth knowing about them, because they were used in a number of important experiments and vector constructions. We will look at a couple of these early methods.

7. 4. 1   Chemical mutagenesis

Some of the methods rely on the chemical modification of bases. One of the most useful reactions involves using bisulphite ions for the deamination of

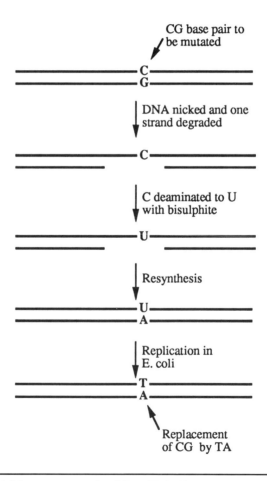

Figure 7.2 **Bisulphite mutagenesis of C to T via U.**

C residues to U residues in single-stranded regions. The procedure is shown in Figure 7.2. One strand of the duplex is degraded over a short region (by nicking and exonuclease treatment; see Section 7.4.3), and the resulting molecule is treated with sodium bisulphite. This converts C residues in the single-stranded region to U residues. The single-stranded region is then converted back to double-stranded with DNA polymerase and dNTPs. The polymerase incorporates A residues opposite the U residues, so that the original CG base pairs will be converted to UA base pairs. The molecules are then reintroduced into a host. The U residue may be replaced with a T residue by the host's DNA repair system (using the enzyme uracil glycosylase), but in any case, subsequent rounds of replication will generate molecules with TA base pairs where formerly there were CG base pairs. This limits the mutagenesis to transition mutations.

7. 4. 2 Enzymatic mutagenesis

It is also possible to rely on DNA polymerase to introduce a point mutation. One method is shown in Figure 7.3 and involves the use of the enzyme to synthesize a short piece of DNA in a single-stranded region in the absence of one nucleotide. The polymerase stalls opposite the complementary base, but misincorporation of one of the other nucleotides may then occur, allowing the second strand to be completed. The double-stranded molecule, which now contains a mismatch, is then introduced into a suitable host. Replication will generate one molecule with the mutated sequence and one with the original sequence. If, on

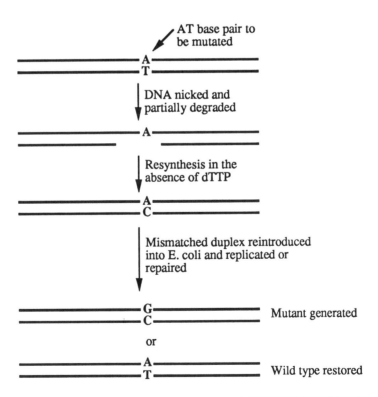

Figure 7.3 **Enzymatic mutagenesis.**

the other hand, the mismatched position is repaired before replication by the normal cellular mismatch-repair systems, the resultant molecule will be either mutant or like the original molecule, depending on the direction of mismatch correction.

7. 4. 3 Generating single-stranded DNA

Both the methods described in Sections 7.4.1 and 7.4.2 require the generation of a small section of single-stranded DNA in the region to be mutated. It may be possible to produce this by cleavage with a restriction enzyme in the presence of ethidium bromide. The intercalated molecule hinders the enzyme, so that only one strand is cut. The nick can then be enlarged by treatment with a suitable exonuclease (according to the direction required) for an appropriate length of time.

7. 5 OLIGONUCLEOTIDE MUTAGENESIS

7. 5. 1 The principles

The early techniques for point mutation presented a number of difficulties – the need to generate a localized region of single-stranded DNA, the need to ascertain the right amount of bisulphite to use, and so on – and use of oligonucleotide-directed mutagenesis rapidly superseded them. The basic technique is summarized in Figure 7.4.

The region to be mutated is cloned into a vector, such as M13, in order to prepare single-stranded DNA. Very often this will be available anyway, from DNA-sequencing studies. An oligonucleotide is synthesized whose sequence contains the mutation but is otherwise complementary to the target DNA. The oligonucleotide is allowed to anneal to the single-stranded DNA, and DNA polymerase and dNTPs are added. The oligonucleotide functions as a primer for the synthesis of the rest of the second strand. The double-stranded molecule is covalently closed with ligase and contains a mismatch at the site of the mutation. It is then reintroduced into *E. coli*. Replication will generate two types of molecule – one with the wild-type and one with the mutated sequence. If mismatch repair takes place before replication, then the molecules will be all wild-type or all mutant, according to the direction of repair. If mismatch repair does not take place and a mixed population of molecules is likely to be present, they must be separated by plaque purification of the phage (repeated plating out of the phage from individual plaques) to generate an entirely homogeneous population. The plaques containing the mutated molecules can be identified by probing with the mutagenic oligonucleotide under stringent conditions, so that the wild-type molecules will not hybridize to it. DNA sequencing, which should be straightforward if the target DNA is already cloned in M13 or an equivalent, is then used to verify that the mutation has occurred and that no other mutations have arisen in the sequence. There are several modifications to this basic approach.

a. More than one site can be mutated at a time by using an oligonucleotide with more than one mismatch to the target sequence.

b. Several different mutations can be made *at the same site* by using an "oligonucleotide" with a mixed site (i.e., a collection of oligonucleotides with different bases at the position in question). Which mutation is made

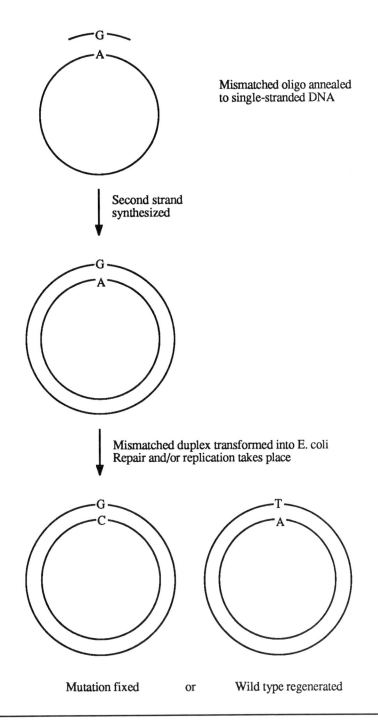

Figure 7.4 **Oligonucleotide mutagenesis: the basic reaction.** The aim is to mutate an A residue in the initial single-stranded molecule to a C.

in any one molecule will depend upon which oligonucleotide from the mixture annealed. After plaque purification, individual phage cultures can be screened by DNA sequencing to verify which mutations have been generated. The use of mixed sites in an oligonucleotide to generate several mutations is often called *cassette mutagenesis*. It is possible to generate large numbers of mutations very quickly this way. For example, an oligonucleotide with two triply mixed sites can generate 15 different mutant sequences (6 single mutations and 9 double mutations).

c. If the target sequence is from a large gene, it is usually preferable to clone a restriction fragment from it into M13 (or an equivalent), mutate that fragment, verify the mutation by sequencing, and then reassemble the gene by replacing the original wild-type restriction fragment with a mutated one. That is because the gene may be too large to clone into M13 in its entirety and because resequencing the entire gene to ensure that only the mutation(s) desired had been generated would be laborious.

7. 5. 2 Improving the efficiency

In the basic technique of oligonucleotide-directed mutagenesis, it would be expected that 50% of the molecules produced would be mutant and 50% would have the original sequence. However, this is often not the case. Some molecules may be able to replicate faster than others, or they may affect host viability differently. Also, mismatch repair might be biased in a particular direction. It may therefore be that the frequency with which mutants are obtained is so low that steps have to be taken to improve it. There are two approaches to improving the efficiency of generating mutants. One is to interfere with the mismatch repair so that the mutant sequence is retained in preference to the original (or is, at any rate, not discriminated against). The other is to apply selection for the mutant sequence. We will deal first with three ways of influencing mismatch repair and then look at how selection can be used.

1. Using *mutS* hosts to stop mismatch repair. We can avoid the possibility that the host's mismatch repair will act against the fixation of the mutation by using a *mutS* host. The *mutS* hosts are deficient in this process, as they lack the MutS protein, which recognizes mismatched regions and binds to them prior to repair. So although there will not be any bias in favour of the mutation when the mismatched duplex is returned into a *mutS* host, at least there will not be any bias against it. A disadvantage with these hosts is that they have an elevated background mutation rate, increasing the chance that extra mutations may take place at other sites in the sequence.

2. Using template containing uracil to bias mismatch repair. To understand this method we must first have some background information on how uracil can become incorporated into DNA and how cells deal with it. Uracil can be formed in DNA by the spontaneous deamination of cytosine, and in a subsequent round of replication, the uracil would direct the incorporation of an A residue on the opposite strand where there had been G initially. The presence of uracil in DNA is therefore potentially mutagenic, and *E. coli* has a mechanism for its removal. This relies on the *ung* gene, encoding a uracil-N-glycosylase. This enzyme removes the uracil from the deoxyribose, leaving an *apyrimidinic site* (i.e., a

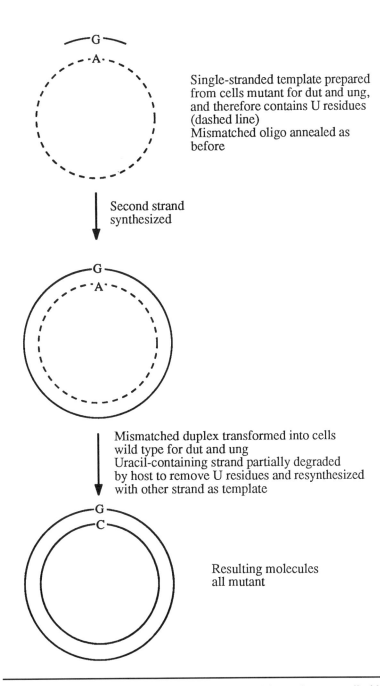

Single-stranded template prepared from cells mutant for dut and ung, and therefore contains U residues (dashed line)
Mismatched oligo annealed as before

Second strand synthesized

Mismatched duplex transformed into cells wild type for dut and ung
Uracil-containing strand partially degraded by host to remove U residues and resynthesized with other strand as template

Resulting molecules all mutant

Figure 7.5 **Mutagenesis using template prepared from** *dut⁻ung⁻* **cells (dashed circle).**

site in which the base is missing but the phosphodiester backbone is intact). The DNA strand containing the apyrimidinic site is then nicked by an endonuclease, and the defective region is degraded and replaced by DNA polymerase I using the other strand as a template. Apart from the deamination of cytosine, U residues can also become incorporated into DNA by the use of dUTP rather than dTTP during replication by DNA polymerase. Cells normally contain only

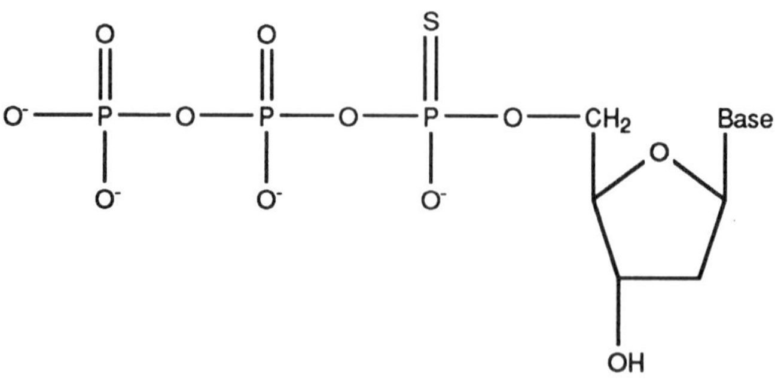

Figure 7.6 **Structure of a phosphorothioate nucleotide.**

low levels of dUTP, which functions as an intermediate in the synthesis of dTTP. The level is kept low by the presence of a dUTPase (catalysing the next step in the synthesis of dTTP) that is the product of the *dut* gene. U that is incorporated into DNA from dUTP will normally be removed in the same way that U arising from C deamination is removed. Cells that are *dut⁻ung⁻* therefore have a high level of uracil in their DNA (in fact, about 1 T in 100 is replaced by U).

These functions of the *dut* and *ung* genes can be exploited in mutagenesis (Figure 7.5). Single-stranded template DNA (containing high levels of U) is prepared from *dut⁻ung⁻* cells. The template is used with the mutagenic oligonucleotide as described before (using dATP, dCTP, dGTP, and dTTP), and the duplex is transformed back into *E. coli*. However, this time the host strain is *ung⁺*, and the activity of the glycosylase and the apyrimidinic-site endonuclease cause widespread degradation of the original template strand, as it contained U residues. The second strand – which of course is the one bearing the mutated sequence – is preserved, as it does not contain U residues. This method has the disadvantage of an increased spontaneous mutation rate in the *dut⁻ung⁻* hosts.

3. Using phosphorothioate nucleotides to bias mismatch repair *in vitro*. It is possible to carry out a form of mismatch repair *in vitro* and bias it using phosphorothioate nucleotide analogues. The general structure of these analogues is shown in Figure 7.6. The replacement of an oxygen atom by a sulphur atom in these nucleotides renders DNA containing such residues resistant to attack by a number of nucleases, including the restriction endonuclease *Nci*I and exonuclease III. This fact is exploited in the following way. The target DNA and mutagenic oligonucleotide are annealed as usual, and the second-strand synthesis is then carried out using at least one phosphorothioate nucleotide. We then treat the DNA with *Nci*I. This cuts the first strand, resulting in nicks, but it cannot cut the second strand because of the presence of phosphorothioate nucleotides in that strand. The nicks in the first strand are then enlarged by treatment with exoIII. The first strand is thus largely degraded. It is then resynthesized by addition of DNA polymerase and dNTPs, using the second strand (which has the mutated sequence) as a template. Both strands will therefore come to have the mutated sequence. The resulting double-stranded material is then reintroduced into a host.

4. Using selection. Positive selection can be used for the mutant strand. This can be done by cloning the target gene in a phagemid that also carries a mutant ampicillin resistance gene (*amp*ˢ, Figure 7.7). Single-stranded template DNA is

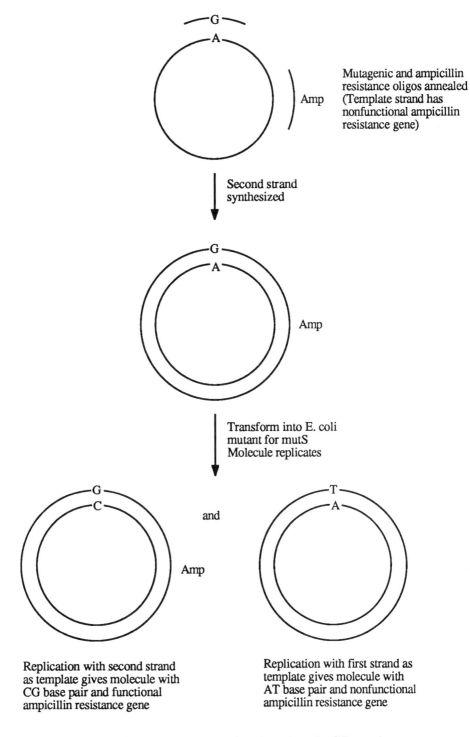

Mutagenic and ampicillin resistance oligos annealed (Template strand has nonfunctional ampicillin resistance gene)

Second strand synthesized

Transform into E. coli mutant for mutS Molecule replicates

and

Replication with second strand as template gives molecule with CG base pair and functional ampicillin resistance gene

Replication with first strand as template gives molecule with AT base pair and nonfunctional ampicillin resistance gene

Selection for ampicillin resistance therefore also selects for CG mutation.

Figure 7.7 Oligonucleotide mutagenesis incorporating selection for mutant molecules.

then prepared and second-strand synthesis carried out. Two mutagenic oligonucleotides are used in the second-strand synthesis. One directs the mutation we are interested in; the other reverts the amp^S to amp^R. After the second-strand synthesis, the template is transformed back into *E. coli*. A *mutS* host is used, so no mismatch correction takes place. Selection for ampicillin resistance allows selection for molecules whose sequence was determined by the amp^R mutagenic oligonucleotide. Because these molecules represent the second strand, whose sequence was determined by the oligonucleotides, they should also have the mutated sequence at the target site. A similar procedure uses a mutant *lacZ* gene instead of the ampicillin resistance one, allowing chromogenic selection rather than direct antibiotic selection. Using two oligonucleotides requires careful control of the annealing conditions, so that as many template molecules as possible have *both* oligonucleotides bound.

7. 5. 3 Mutagenesis by PCR

PCR can be used in site-directed mutagenesis, as described in Section 6.2.3.

7. 6 CHOOSING THE RIGHT MUTATIONS

The most important aspect of any site-directed mutagenesis project is not the generation of the mutants, which ought to be straightforward, but deciding which mutations to make. Careful consideration must be given not only to which nucleotide to mutate, but what it should be mutated to. To do this properly requires detailed knowledge of the function of the target sequence. If the sequence encodes a protein, then some idea of the protein's structure and of the residues that are important for function is usually necessary. Ideally, the three-dimensional structure of the molecule would be known, although this is rarely the case. It is also important to realize that minor changes in amino acid sequence can have a profound effect on the overall three-dimensional structure, perhaps even abolishing activity, even though there may be no change in the primary sequence at the active site. Computer modelling may allow prediction of the effects of particular mutations on the three-dimensional structure; changes may also be detected by spectroscopic analysis of either nuclear magnetic resonance or circular dichroism, or by looking at antibody binding and protease resistance (which may be reduced in proteins that have not folded correctly).

7. 7 INACTIVATING GENES

It is often useful to inactivate endogenous genes in an organism. This might help us to find out the physiological role of the wild-type gene; to allow the expression of a mutated gene (produced by the means described in Section 7.5) in the absence of a background of expression of the wild-type gene; or, in a biotechnological setting, to inactivate an undesirable gene. There are three ways in which inactivation can most conveniently be achieved. One involves the disruption of the DNA sequence; the other two involve the inactivation of the relevant RNA. The vectors, transformation systems, and so on, that are used depend on the organism involved (see Chapter 9), but the principles are largely the same and will be presented here. Note that before trying to inactivate a gene – whatever method is used – it is important to consider whether the result is likely to be lethal to the organism. If it is, the technique will always appear to fail, since no gene-inactivated individuals will be recovered as they are all dead!

7.7.1 Gene disruption

The principle of gene disruption is to use homologous recombination to replace the endogenous chromosomal copy of a gene with an inactivated copy. The procedure is shown in Figure 7.8. The gene to be disrupted is cloned, and a selectable marker – perhaps an antibiotic resistance or a nutritional marker – is introduced into it. Insertion of the selectable marker must render the target gene nonfunctional, and it may be necessary to verify that this will indeed be the case. The disrupted gene is then excised from its vector (or at least the construct is linearized), and the linear DNA is introduced into the target organism. Selection is then imposed for the inserted antibiotic resistance or nutritional marker. The incoming molecule bearing the marker will not be stably replicated, as the molecule is linear. Stable acquisition of the marker can take place only if a double crossover across the flanking sequences and their chromosomal counterparts causes the marker's integration into the chromosome, replacing the endogenous chromosomal copy of the gene by the disrupted one. So individuals that have stably acquired the marker should have had the chromosomal copy of the target gene replaced by the disrupted copy.

Apart from the general problem of lethality discussed in the opening of Section 7.7, gene disruption has certain other limitations. If the target organism normally contains more than one copy of the gene, it may be difficult to ensure that all copies are disrupted. This is especially true if the selectable marker is dominant (which is normally the case), since one copy of the marker will have the same effect as several. Multiple copies of the gene are likely to be present if the organism is not haploid or if there are several copies of the gene per haploid genome (i.e., the gene is part of a multigene family). An efficient homologous recombination system is necessary to direct integration of the disrupted gene copy at the site of the endogenous gene, rather than elsewhere in the genome. Gene disruption is widely used in bacteria, yeast, and animals. The particular

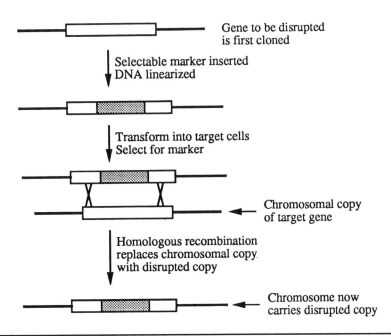

Figure 7.8 **Gene disruption**. Replacement with a disrupted copy.

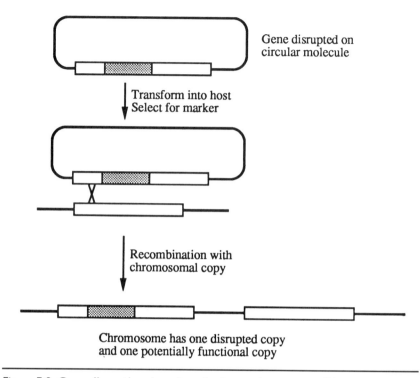

Figure 7.9 Gene disruption. Insertion of a disrupted copy may still leave a functional copy in the chromosome.

problems posed by the need for homologous recombination in mammalian systems are discussed in Section 9.9.3.

It is not always necessary to supply the disrupting copy on a linear molecule. It can be supplied on a circular molecule, provided this is unable to replicate in the host used and can be stably maintained only by chromosomal integration. In this case, a single crossover is sufficient for integration, but the disrupting copy needs to have been inactivated by more than just the insertion of a selectable marker (e.g., by truncation); otherwise, the recombination and integration will reconstitute a functional gene (composed of part of the disrupting sequence and part of the chromosomal copy), as shown in Figure 7.9. Integration of a molecule in this way can be exploited to disrupt the endogenous copy of a gene and to insert an altered – but functional – one.

7. 7. 2 Antisense sequences

The synthesis in a cell of an RNA molecule with a sequence that is complementary to another RNA molecule can interfere with the function of the latter – either by simple base-pairing between the RNAs or by some more subtle process. This effect is used physiologically – for example, in the control of replication of certain *E. coli* plasmids. In artificial manipulations, a DNA sequence encoding an RNA complementary to the RNA to be inactivated (an *antisense RNA*) is placed under the control of a suitable, powerful promoter and inserted into the organism of interest. Expression from the promoter then generates antisense RNA, and the level of expression of the endogenous gene is diminished. It is difficult to get complete inactivation this way, in contrast to the consequences of gene disruption, but levels of expression can be reduced to a few percent or less of wild type. The technique does not suffer so much from the drawbacks of the gene disruption method (need for homologous recombination, problems of multiple gene copies, etc.) mentioned in Section 7.7.1. The antisense RNA approach has been particularly successfully used with plants (see Section 9.6.7). The exact mechanism for suppression of gene expression is not clear. It is possible that the antisense RNA forms a duplex with the mRNA in the cytoplasm, and the duplex cannot be translated (perhaps because it is broken down by double-strand-specific ribonucleases). However, it is also possible that the inactivation takes place earlier, within the nucleus – perhaps as a result of interference with RNA processing. Gene expression can also be reduced by using antisense oligonucleotides, rather than antisense RNA. In this case, the oligonucleotides are introduced directly into the target cells.

An unexpected observation with antisense RNA work was *cosuppression*. This is the down-regulation of expression of endogenous genes by transformation with constructs intended to generate *sense* RNA, rather than *antisense* RNA. The mechanism is not clear, but it has been suggested that the phenomenon is caused by the production of antisense RNA from the constructs, by readthrough from endogenous promoters located near the site of the insertion of DNA into the genome. Other causes, such as methylation of the endogenous gene, have also been suggested.

7.7.3 Ribozymes

In some circumstances, RNA molecules can have direct catalytic activity, such as the removal of certain introns from RNA by self-splicing. The term *ribozyme* is sometimes used to describe any sort of RNA molecule that shows catalytic activity. However, the term is sometimes used more specifically to refer to RNA molecules that carry out a self-cleavage reaction, and these are the examples we consider here. Most of the examples come from RNAs that are associated with plant pathogenic viruses and viroids, such as the tobacco ringspot virus or the avocado sunblotch viroid. However, similar instances have also been reported from a few other systems, such as the hepatitis delta virus (which is usually associated with hepatitis B virus). The reaction catalysed is an internal nucleophilic attack by a 2'-hydroxyl of the RNA on the phosphate group of the sugar-phosphate chain at the cleavage site. Because it involves the 2'-hydroxyl, this reaction is necessarily confined to RNA rather than DNA. *In vivo*, this reaction is probably used to cleave into monomers molecules that are produced as concatemers by a rolling circle mechanism; the monomers are subsequently turned into circular monomers by ligation. The sequence requirements for the cleavage are relatively few, but they are always found within a region that is capable of forming a "hammerhead" structure. Figure 7.10 illustrates this structure and also indicates the cleavage site. It is possible for the substrate molecule to be a separate one from the rest of the hammerhead, as long as the correct base-pairing can form. In other words, the sequence requirements for the substrate molecule are very small indeed; therefore, if we know the sequence of a given RNA molecule, we should be able to tailor a catalytic molecule that can form a hammerhead with the first molecule and cleave it. A

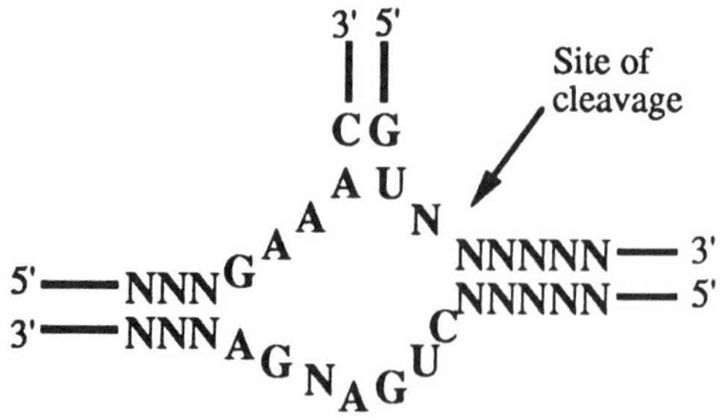

Figure 7.10 **Ribozyme self-cleavage.** Cleavage takes place within the "hammerhead" structure shown. The sequence requirements for the cleaved molecule are minimal.

gene that will direct the synthesis of this catalytic molecule can therefore be constructed and introduced into a host organism, and any suitable substrate RNA molecule should therefore be cleaved. Although there has been considerable success in demonstrating ribozyme-mediated cleavage *in vitro*, success *in vivo* has been more restricted, and it is often difficult to show unambiguously that a given RNA has been inactivated by ribozyme-mediated cleavage rather than by a simple antisense-RNA reaction. Nevertheless, there is considerable interest in this technology, particularly as a way of inactivating intracellular pathogens such as viruses.

CHAPTER

8

Use of Cloned DNA

8. 1 As DNA

There are many uses for particular cloned pieces of DNA as DNA, rather than
as a way of making RNA or protein. We saw in Section 3.2.3 how DNA can be
sequenced and that there are several vector systems designed specifically with
this aim in mind. The other ways of using DNA directly, which generally do not
rely on specialized cloning systems, are too numerous to describe here in depth.
They include blotting (Southern, Northern, Southwestern, etc.), transcript mapping, footprinting, and bandshift assaying, and details of these can be found in
general molecular and cell biology textbooks. We will concentrate in this chapter on the use of cloned DNA sequences for *expression* or, in other words, for
directing the synthesis of RNA or protein. As we shall see, many cloning vectors have been developed specifically for this purpose. They are called *expression vectors*.

8. 2 SYNTHESIS OF RNA

8. 2. 1 Why synthesize RNA?

It may be necessary to produce RNA for a number of reasons. We might be
studying autocatalytic splicing or cleavage events and need to produce RNA of

a single type in the presence of as few contaminating proteins as possible. Or the aim might be to make a protein in a radiolabelled form by translation *in vitro* of an appropriate RNA in the presence of radioactive amino acids.

8. 2. 2   Vector systems

One approach to making RNA might be to use a vector with a powerful promoter to direct transcription in a bacterial cell *in vivo*, and then isolate the RNA. However, because the purification of RNA from bacterial cells is difficult, and the isolation of individual RNA species even more so, the production of RNA is usually done by transcription from cloned DNA *in vitro*. The most widely used systems utilize promoters from the bacteriophages T7 and SP6, but T3 promoters are also used. These phages encode novel RNA polymerases that are synthesized after infection of *E. coli* and that are very specific for phage promoters (see Section 1.3.2). A typical example of one of these vectors is illustrated in Figure 8.1. The vectors contain both T7 and SP6 promoters, oriented to direct transcription into the multiple cloning site that separates them. So it is always possible to transcribe a cloned sequence – regardless of the orientation in which it is cloned – by selecting the appropriate polymerase to activate the appropriate promoter. Transcription from the other promoter may be used to generate an antisense-strand RNA.

All that is necessary for transcription is the incubation of the plasmid DNA *in vitro* with the appropriate polymerase and other substrates. Capping of the message can be achieved, if necessary, by incubation of the transcripts with the cap-

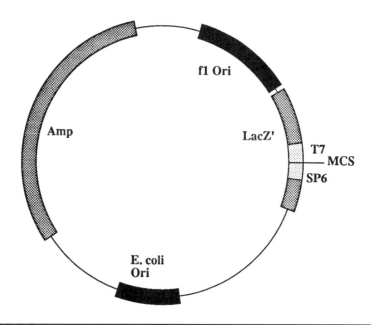

Figure 8.1 **pGEM11Zf (3.2 kb).** The vector contains a selectable ampicillin resistance gene (Amp), origins of replication for double-stranded (E. coli Ori) or single-stranded (f1 Ori) DNA synthesis, and a multiple cloning site (MCS) in a lacZ' gene. The MCS is flanked by T7 and SP6 promoters, allowing transcription *in vitro* of sequences inserted in either orientation.

ping enzyme guanylyl transferase and GTP. If the first nucleotide to be incorporated into the transcript is a G, then it may be possible to bring about capping during transcription by the inclusion in the reaction of a cap analogue, G(5')ppp(5')G, in excess over the normal nucleotide ppp(5')G. The cap analogue can be incorporated only at the beginning of the transcript (because the 5' groups, which would be needed for incorporation elsewhere, are in effect blocked by each other), but it will necessarily be incorporated at the beginning because it is in excess over GTP. If it is important to avoid any transcription beyond the insert into the vector sequences, then the plasmid can be linearized by digestion with an appropriate restriction enzyme (cutting just beyond the site of insert integration) prior to transcription *in vitro*. Note that the example in Figure 8.1 has the site of insertion within a section of the *lacZ* gene, and therefore, as described earlier, we can verify the presence or absence of insert by the colony colour on plates containing X-Gal. The plasmid also contains the filamentous phage f1 replication origin, so that if cells containing the plasmid are subsequently infected with an appropriate helper phage, single-stranded DNA can be produced, packaged, and secreted into the medium. This may be helpful for checking the sequence of what has been inserted into the multiple cloning site.

8. 3 SYNTHESIS OF PROTEIN

8. 3. 1 Why synthesize protein?

It is extremely common to need to express cloned genes so we can make the proteins they encode. We may need to prepare small quantities of radiolabelled proteins, perhaps for studies on co- or posttranslational targeting or modification of proteins. Alternatively, we may want to produce larger amounts of the protein in a nonradioactive form, perhaps as a prelude to purification for determination of some of its properties in biological or biochemical assays, or perhaps to crystallize it for structural studies. Or we may want to prepare an altered protein after site-directed mutagenesis to ascertain the consequences that the mutations we have generated have for the catalytic properties of an enzyme.

8. 3. 2 The problems encountered

If we simply need to prepare small quantities of a radiolabelled protein, this is usually most easily accomplished by translation *in vitro* of RNA produced by transcription *in vitro* (see Section 8.2.2). This is generally relatively straightforward. Occasionally, translation of small quantities of RNA is carried out *in vivo*; for example, by microinjection into *Xenopus* oocytes. Larger quantities of proteins are usually prepared by transcription and translation *in vivo*, and there are a number of problems to overcome with these procedures. We need to consider the following:

    a. transcription and translation initiation

    b. fate of the transcript

    c. efficiency of translation

    d. fate of the protein after synthesis

Methods for dealing with these considerations depend on the vectors used.

8. 3. 3 Translation *in vitro*

There are three common methods of directing protein synthesis *in vitro*. The two most commonly used employ a reticulocyte lysate or a wheat germ extract. The reticulocyte lysate comes from rabbits. Reticulocytes are prepared and lysed, and the extract is treated with micrococcal nuclease. This degrades the endogenous mRNA in the extract, which otherwise would produce a high background of translation products. The extract is then treated with EGTA, which chelates the calcium ions needed for the functioning of the micrococcal nuclease. If the nuclease is not inactivated, the added mRNA will be degraded. Instead, added mRNA will be translated, and if a radioactive amino acid (or acids) is included (usually methionine – although others, such as cysteine and leucine, are also frequently used), the protein produced will be radioactive. The second commonly used system for directing protein synthesis *in vitro* is an extract of wheat germ cells. Basically, this is prepared by grinding wheat germ in a suitable buffer, removing cell debris, and treating with micrococcal nuclease followed by EGTA as with the reticulocyte lysate.

The third method for translation *in vitro* uses an "S-30" extract of *E. coli* cells. Cells of a suitable strain (usually one deficient in RNase activity) are lysed, and the supernatant of a 30,000 g centrifuge spin is taken. This is the S-30 extract. It contains ribosomes and the other components of the protein synthesis machinery, but it does not contain the DNA, which was pelleted. Many of the ribosomes will be in the process of translating mRNA, so the extract is preincubated to allow the completion of translation that has already been initiated. In prokaryotes, transcription and translation are usually coupled; that is, translation of the RNA is initiated while RNA is still being produced by transcription. Consequently, once translation of endogenous RNA is completed, it will not be reinitiated. Also, any fully transcribed RNA that is added to the system will not be translated efficiently. So rather than transcribe RNA separately and then add it to the S-30 extract as we would do with the reticulocyte lysate or wheat germ systems, we add DNA to the extract. Remember that the extract contains the machinery for transcription as well as translation. Any genes that have a promoter recognized by the S-30 extract (i.e., a typical *E. coli* one) can therefore be transcribed and translated. As with the other systems, a radioactive amino acid is supplied, and radiolabelled protein is produced.

8. 3. 4 Transcription and translation *in vivo*

1. Transcription and translation initiation. It is often not enough simply to attach the coding sequence we want to express to a powerful, unregulated promoter and ribosome binding site, as many proteins are toxic to *E. coli* cells when overexpressed in this way. If the overexpressed protein is toxic, no colonies will be recovered after transformation with the recombinant plasmid, because any transformed cells will be killed by the overexpression of the protein. It is possible that a few colonies might be recovered, with mutations in the cloned gene that either abolish the gene's expression or modify the characteristics of the protein produced so that it is no longer toxic (but – in addition – no longer the protein that we are interested in). So it is usually preferable to use a powerful, but controllable, promoter.

As well as directing *transcription* initiation, we need to direct *translation* initiation. In *E. coli*, this is done by a ribosome binding site. This is composed

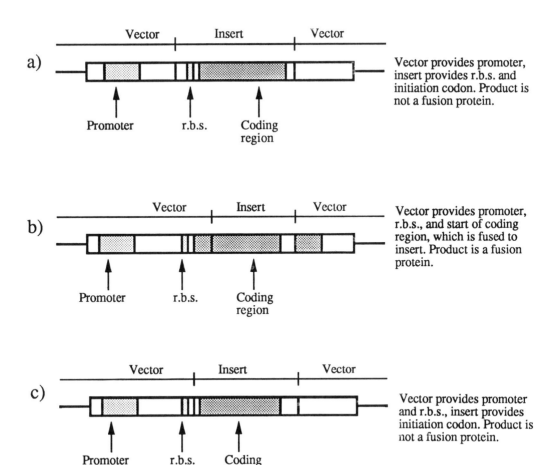

Figure 8.2 **Expression of cloned sequences.** r.b.s. = ribosome binding site.

of a sequence of a few nucleotides in the mRNA, typically -GAGG-, shortly before the translation initiation codon. It is complementary to a few nucleotides at the 3' end of the *E. coli* 16S rRNA. That sequence allows the small subunit of the ribosome to bind to the mRNA by complementary base-pairing. Translation starts at the first AUG codon in the mRNA downstream from the ribosome binding site. If the sequence inserted into the vector contains its own ribosome binding site, there is no need for one to be supplied by the vector (Figure 8.2a). If the inserted sequence does not contain a ribosome binding site, though, the vector must provide it. There are two ways of using a vector to do this.

One way is to generate a *fusion protein* (Figure 8.2b). To do this, the vector contains, downstream from the promoter, a ribosome binding site followed by the initiation codon and coding region for a protein. Sequences are inserted into this coding region. The inserted sequence has no nontranslated information. The reading frame in the vector is in phase with the insert and runs directly into it. Translation runs directly from the vector coding region into the insert coding region, and the result is a fusion protein that has vector-encoded sequence at its N-terminus, and insert-encoded sequence at its C-terminus. As we will see, there are ways of removing this vector-encoded protein quite specifically.

The other way of getting the vector to provide the translation initiation signal is simply to have a ribosome binding site immediately preceding the cloning site (Figure 8.2c). Translation will start at the first AUG in the inserted sequence (provided that it is not more than a few nucleotides from the ribosome binding site in the vector).

We will now look at the most commonly used expression systems.

*LAC*Z PROMOTER. We have already come across one example of a powerful controllable promoter. This is the promoter of the *lacZ* gene, contained in the pUC and M13 vectors and in the lambda ZAP and Bluescript series. The promoter is controlled by the LacI repressor. This is often encoded in the vector, or it can be furnished by the host. In the presence of IPTG, the repressor function is inactivated, and expression from the promoter occurs. Sequences inserted into the multiple cloning site in the *lacZ* gene in these vectors will then be expressed. Translation can be from any suitable ribosome binding sites on the inserted DNA, or as a fusion protein with the *lacZ* sequence, provided the inserted DNA is in the right reading frame. The fact that the inserted DNA can be expressed is particularly useful for immunochemical screening of libraries, which was described in Section 5.2.2. A difficulty may arise where the vector under consideration is present in the cell at a high copy number, and the repressor gene is present on an F' plasmid at a much lower copy number. The multiple copies of the vector may be sufficient to titrate out all the repressor and allow expression in the absence of inducer. This problem of unwanted expression can be largely avoided by use of the *lacI*^{q} allele of the repressor. This carries a mutation in the promoter for the repressor itself, resulting in about 10-fold higher levels of repressor per cell than are obtained with the wild-type repressor allele. In many vectors the lac repressor gene is carried on the vector molecule itself, which also helps to increase the amount of repressor in the cell and allows greater flexibility in the choice of host strain.

LAMBDA. The powerful leftward promoter (P_L) of bacteriophage lambda is tightly controlled by the lambda CI repressor protein. The pP$_L$-lambda vector shown in Figure 8.3 contains this promoter. Sequences are inserted in the *N* gene (which is also part of the region derived from bacteriophage lambda) at the *Hpa*I site. Control of the promoter via the operator (O_L) is achieved using a

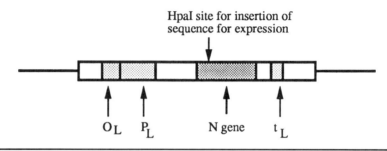

Figure 8.3 Expression region of the pP$_L$-lambda vector (5.2 kb). The vector also contains an origin of replication and an ampicillin resistance selectable marker.

suitable host. Perhaps the easiest way is to use a host that produces a mutant CI repressor protein (CI^{857}) that is temperature sensitive. At 30°C or lower, the repressor produced by the host is active, and the promoter is kept under repression. Raising the temperature inactivates the repressor, and the promoter is activated. Another way of activating the promoter is to add nalidixic acid to the growth medium. This inhibits DNA gyrase and causes induction of synthesis of the *E. coli* RecA protein. The RecA protein causes cleavage of the lambda repressor and consequent activation of the promoter. Translation with the pP$_L$-lambda vector requires either that the insert provides its own ribosome binding site or that the insert directs production of a fusion protein with the *N* gene product. There is a transcription terminator (t$_L$) to avoid transcription reading through and interfering with other plasmid functions. In some lambda-based vectors, fusion with the *cII* gene is used.

T7 PROMOTERS. Some systems use expression from a T7 phage promoter *in vivo*. To provide the T7 polymerase, the gene for it is present also (either on the vector itself or in a coresident plasmid in the host) and is controlled by another promoter, such as that for *lacZ*.

HYBRIDS. A number of powerful promoters have been constructed artificially as hybrids between existing promoters. The vector pKK223-3 (Figure 8.4) contains one of these hybrids. The promoter is called the *tac* promoter and is a hybrid between the -35 region of the promoter of the *trp* operon and the -10 region of the *lac* promoter (actually, the *lac*UV5 promoter – a form with two mutations in the -10 region, which result in enhanced expression). The *tac* promoter includes the *lac* operator and is regulated by the lac repressor, which has to be supplied by the host. Transcription is induced by addition of IPTG to the medium. Beyond the *tac* promoter is a multiple cloning site, where sequences can be inserted (Figure 8.5a). Depending on the restriction site used, expression will be from a ribosome binding site in the plasmid close to the multiple cloning site, or the insert may need to provide a ribosome binding site. Beyond the multiple cloning site is a powerful transcription terminator (and the 5S rRNA gene, which is not necessary for expression purposes but was inserted along with the terminator) from the *E. coli rrnB* rRNA operon. Active transcription of the whole plasmid can interfere with replication, so the incorporation of this terminator helps to improve plasmid stability. A relative of this plasmid, pKK233-2,

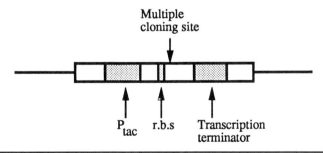

Multiple
cloning site

P$_{tac}$ r.b.s   Transcription
terminator

Figure 8.4 **Expression region of the pKK223-3 vector (4.6 kb).** The vector also contains an origin of replication and an ampicillin resistance selectable marker.

AGG<u>AAACAGA</u><u>ATTCCCGGG</u><u>GGATCC</u>GTCGAC<u>CTGCAG</u>CC<u>AAGCTT</u>   pKK223-3
r.b.s.   EcoRI   BamHI   PstI   HindIII

                    SmaI   SalI
                    XmaI   AccI
a)   HincII

AGG<u>AAACAGA</u><u>CCATGG</u>CTGCAGCC<u>AAGCTT</u>   pKK233-2
r.b.s.   NcoI   ___   HindIII
b)   PstI

Figure 8.5 **Multiple cloning site of the plasmids pKK223-3 (upper) and pKK233-2 (lower).** Note the ribosome binding sites upstream from both multiple cloning sites, and the potential ATG codon in pKK233-2.

has the *trc* promoter, which differs from the *tac* promoter by having the -10 and -35 sequences one nucleotide farther apart. This causes a slight reduction in promoter activity. The cloning site has a sequence (Figure 8.5b) that places a *Nco*I site containing ATG just beyond the ribosome binding site, followed by a *Pst*I site and a *Hin*dIII site. This arrangement facilitates expression of inserted sequences using the ribosome binding site and initiation codon of the vector.

Controllable promoters are also available as *cassettes* – fragments with a range of restriction sites that can conveniently be inserted adjacent to the coding region of interest.

2. Dealing with fusion proteins. When expression *in vivo* generates a fusion protein, it is likely to be difficult to separate the vector-encoded part of the protein from the insert-encoded region that is of more interest. However, a number of vectors are available that allow this to be done. In these vectors, the junction between the vector-encoded part of the fusion and the insert-encoded part is engineered to be the recognition site for a specific protease. An example of this, pGEX-3X, is given in Figure 8.6. This vector produces a fusion protein with glutathione S-transferase (under the control of the *tac* promoter). The junction between the vector sequence and the site of insertion of DNA for expression encodes the sequence -Ile-Glu-Gly-Arg-, which is the recognition site for Factor Xa, one of the specific proteases involved in activating the blood clotting pathway. A similar example, pGEX-2T (Figure 8.6), has the recognition site for thrombin (-Leu-Val-Pro-Arg-Gly-Ser-) encoded at the junction.

The production of the protein of interest as part of a fusion with some other well-characterized protein may have advantages when it comes to purifying the overexpressed protein, particularly if it is easy to purify the vector-encoded part of the fusion. For example, in the case of pGEX-3X, the glutathione S-transferase part of the protein has a high affinity for glutathione. The fusion protein can therefore be recovered from a cell extract by passing the extract through a column of glutathione attached to a suitable support, such as Sepharose 4-B. Passing free glutathione through the column then allows elution of the bound

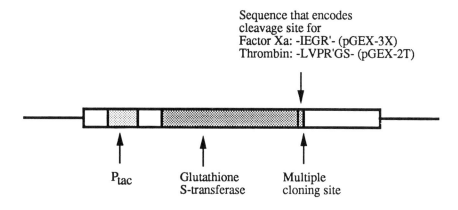

Figure 8.6 Expression regions of the plasmids pGEX-3X and pGEX-2T (4.9 kb). The vectors also have an origin of replication, an ampicillin resistance selectable marker, and a *lacI*q gene to supply repressor for control of the *tac* promoter. The vectors differ in the cleavage site that is encoded adjacent to the multiple cloning site.

fusion protein (by equilibration of the fusion protein between the glutathione-Sepharose and the free glutathione). Fusion constructs with beta-galactosidase can similarly be purified by passage through a column containing beta-galactosidase antibodies or containing a covalently bound, noncleavable beta-galactosidase substrate analogue, such as p-aminophenyl-ß-D-thiogalactosidyl-succinyldiamino-hexyl-Sepharose. Release from the column can be arranged by disrupting antibody-antigen interaction or by passing free substrate through the column. Alternatively, if a fusion protein has a proteolytic cleavage site at the junction, the desired protein can be released by passage of the protease through the column.

A modification of the fusion protein approach for protein purification involves engineering several (often five) histidine codons onto the 3' end of the coding sequence to be expressed. The resulting polyhistidine stretch at the C-terminus of the protein can be used for affinity purification on columns with immobilized cations such as nickel, copper, or zinc. These form strong complexes with the polyhistidine tails. Elution from the column can be achieved with a pH gradient or EDTA, and the polyhistidine tail removed (if necessary) with carboxypeptidase.

3. Fate of the transcript. A considerable amount of modification of the coding region of RNA molecules can take place in eukaryotes before translation. Most notable is the excision of introns, but other reactions can take place too, such as the deletion and insertion of individual residues (*editing*). In general, these processes do not take place in *E. coli* (although introns are not completely absent from prokaryotes), and genes that would normally require processing of their transcripts will not be expressed. The need for processing can be circumvented by expressing a cDNA molecule, rather than the gene itself. Assuming this cDNA has been generated from the fully processed message, there will be no need for further processing of transcripts generated from it.

4. Efficiency of translation. Assuming transcription and translation can be initiated efficiently, it cannot be assumed that the rest of translation will be efficient. Factors that may influence the efficiency of expression are codon usage, codon meaning, and the presence of introns (see "Fate of the transcript" earlier in Section 8.3.4).

Most amino acids can be encoded by a number of different codons, and not all codons are used equally frequently. Likewise, the tRNAs that recognize them vary in abundance. There may be differences in codon preference from one gene to another both within the same organism and between organisms. If the gene that is to be expressed contains many codons whose corresponding tRNA is present only at low abundance, the overall rate of synthesis of the protein may be low, because the codons are read only with low efficiency. If we use site-directed mutagenesis to substitute for the offending codons ones that are read more efficiently, that may relieve the problem.

The genetic code is not universal, although deviations from it are relatively uncommon. However, if the gene we want to express comes from a system where the code is different, then expression in a system using the universal code is likely to lead to an altered product. This is perhaps most easily seen for those mitochondria (such as mammalian ones) that use UGA as a tryptophan codon, rather than a stop codon. Expression of a gene containing UGA tryptophan codons in *E. coli* will lead to the formation of a truncated polypeptide, because the UGA codons are read as stop codons and protein synthesis is thereby terminated. To avoid this, site-directed mutagenesis can be used to change the UGA codons to UGG codons. Alternatively, one could make use of a "chain-termination suppressor" strain of *E. coli*. Such strains contain mutated tRNA genes whose products have anticodons that are complementary to one of the termination codons. They can therefore "read" a stop codon as something else and, in this particular example, the UGA could be read as a tryptophan codon in an appropriate host. Because protein-coding regions frequently terminate with more than one type of termination codon, the end of the protein should be unaffected.

5. Fate of the protein after synthesis. The yield of a protein is not determined simply by the rate of synthesis. It also depends on the stability of the protein after synthesis. Even if the protein is synthesized at a high rate, the yield will be low if the protein is rapidly broken down. It is also important to consider where the protein will end up – if it will remain soluble in the cytoplasm, form an insoluble aggregate, enter the cytoplasmic membrane, or pass through it into the periplasm – and whether any modification of the protein is needed for biological activity.

STABILITY. Very often, foreign proteins that are expressed at high levels form insoluble inclusion bodies inside cells. This seems to be particularly likely for proteins expressed as fusions with the *trpE* and *cII* genes, and, although subsequent purification of the proteins may be facilitated, solubilization without destroying biological activity may be difficult. However, the insolubility may help to protect against degradation, which often affects foreign proteins in *E. coli*. Why this degradation should occur is not completely clear. It may be that if the protein concerned normally forms a complex with others, it is unable to form a correctly folded structure in their absence. This results in partial denaturation and increased protease susceptibility.

The degradation of foreign proteins within *E. coli* cells appears to depend largely on ATP-dependent proteases, and one of the major ones is the product of the *lon* gene. This protease is apparently particularly active against partially or completely denatured proteins. Inactivation of the *lon* gene can therefore be used to reduce the degradation of foreign proteins. This causes further difficulties, though, because the *lon* mutation can confer undesirable properties on the host cells. These include mucoidy and UV sensitivity, and sometimes reduced plasmid stability and transformation efficiency. Mucoidy is caused by overproduction of the polysaccharide capsule of the cells and makes them difficult to manipulate physically. Mucoidy can, however, be suppressed by an additional mutation. This is often a mutation in the *galE* gene, or in the *cpsA–E* gene cluster (all of which are needed for synthesis of capsule polysaccharide). The tendency to mucoidy can also be reduced by alteration of the growth conditions, such as use of rich media and growth temperatures above 37°C.

Another protease which can lead to degradation of foreign proteins is the product of the *clpA* gene. Mutations in this are particularly useful in a background that is already *lon⁻*. A number of proteases are under the control of the *htpR* heat-shock response gene, so mutations in this may also be helpful.

DESTINATION. Secretion of a protein from the cell into the periplasmic space – or even into the growth medium – after synthesis, may help to protect against proteolysis and will facilitate subsequent purification. Secretion may also aid in the formation of disulphide bridges, which form less readily within the cytoplasm. The formation of such bridges may not necessarily be an advantage, of course, depending on whether they are found in the protein in its functional state. Secretion generally (but not always) requires the presence of an N-terminal

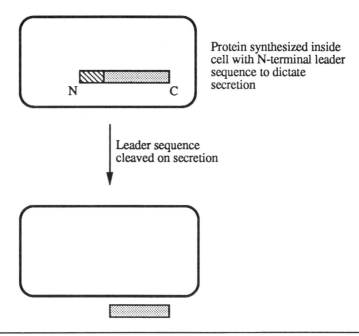

Figure 8.7 **Secretion of a protein dictated by a cleavable N-terminal leader sequence.**

leader sequence on a protein, which is subsequently removed by a leader peptidase. In addition, for some proteins, sequences within the mature protein itself may have important effects on the efficiency of secretion. To direct the secretion of a foreign protein, we therefore usually arrange for it to be synthesized as a fusion with the leader sequence of a secreted protein (Figure 8.7). Leader sequences of *E. coli* proteins that have been used in this way include those of beta-lactamase, the outer membrane proteins OmpA and OmpF, PhoA (alkaline phosphatase), and the filamentous phage gene III protein. It is also possible to use leader sequences of genes from other bacteria, such as the PelB protein from *Erwinia carotovora,* a pectate lyase that functions naturally in the breakdown of plant cell walls. Protein can also be exported from a cell as part of a fully formed phage, as in the phage display vectors described in Section 3.2.4. In general, secretion of proteins from *E. coli* is not always reliable, and other species, such as *Bacillus subtilis,* may be more suitable (see Section 9.3.4).

MODIFICATION. Many eukaryotic proteins require modifications, such as glycosylation, for biological activity. In general, prokaryotic expression systems will be unable to make these modifications, and it is then necessary to use one of the eukaryotic systems discussed in Chapter 9.

6. Other factors. There are other factors that may be important in maximizing expression from a particular gene, particularly in industrial contexts. They include vector copy number and stability. Many of these factors are not well understood, and for most routine laboratory work are secondary considerations. There are plasmids available whose copy number can be controlled. They generally work by regulating the synthesis of a specific primer needed for replication. If the region encoding the primer is placed under a suitably controllable promoter, regulation of replication and thence copy number can be achieved.

CHAPTER

9

Using Other Organisms

9.1 INTRODUCTION

So far, we have concentrated on the techniques for modifying the genome of *E. coli*. However, it is very likely that we need to work with other organisms, too. We might want to make genetically altered versions of commercially important species, such as crop plants, to improve their value. Or we might want to produce a protein in a form that requires some posttranslational modification that *E. coli* was unable to accomplish. The principles that we have seen for *E. coli* apply in exactly the same way. We need to have means of getting the DNA into the organism, suitable vectors, and a means of selecting transformants. We may also need to take steps to increase expression. Often, we first clone DNA from one organism in *E. coli* and identify a recombinant containing a particular gene of interest. We then transfer that gene into some other host species to alter its properties. An organism containing a gene derived from elsewhere is said to be *transgenic*.

In this chapter we will look at the transformation systems for other organisms and the types of vectors available. We will look at Gram-negative bacteria, Gram-positive bacteria, fungi, plants, and animals. Rather than giving a detailed listing of all the methodologies for all the organisms – details of which can be found in primary research papers, reviews, and laboratory manuals – we will concentrate on a representative sample of organisms to look at how the principles we have already encountered can be applied.

9. 2 GRAM-NEGATIVE BACTERIA

We have already looked in detail at one Gram-negative bacterium, *E. coli*. A number of Gram-negative bacteria are also of particular interest for genetic manipulation. They include *Agrobacterium rhizogenes* and *Agrobacterium tumefaciens*, plant pathogens of special importance for the genetic manipulation of plants (described in Section 9.6.1); other plant pathogens, such as *Erwinia carotovora*; a number of human pathogens, such as *Salmonella typhimurium* and *Campylobacter jejuni*; and photosynthetic bacteria, such as the cyanobacteria (significant both as model systems for studying plant photosynthesis and for the ability that some have to fix nitrogen).

9. 2. 1 Transformation systems and hosts

There are three major ways of introducing foreign DNA into cells. These are chemically induced competence (e.g., by treatment with calcium chloride), electroporation, and conjugal transfer (that is, transfer from another species, such as *E. coli*, by conjugation). We have already dealt with the first two treatments in Section 2.2. In conjugation, two cells become physically linked by a proteinaceous tube (or *pilus*), and DNA is passed from one cell to the other. This is how the F (for "fertility") plasmid, which forms the basis of a lot of classical *E. coli* genetics, is transferred from one cell to another. The F factor encodes all the functions necessary for its own transfer. However, other, smaller, plasmids exist that are more suitable for artificial transfer between species. The plasmid to be transferred (sometimes called the *cargo* plasmid) is often unable to direct its own transfer. Instead, it relies on a *conjugal* plasmid that is able to do so, and sometimes also on one or more *helper* plasmids that may encode functions such as methylases that will protect the cargo from degradation in its future host. The helper plasmid may also carry functions needed for the transfer of the cargo. The transfer is achieved in a triparental mating (Figure 9.1), of the following three conjugants: *E. coli* carrying the conjugal plasmid; *E. coli* carrying the cargo and any helper plasmids; and the recipient bacterial species to be manipulated. Conjugation between the the two strains of *E. coli* places all the plasmids necessary in one *E. coli* cell, and conjugation with the recipient bacterium transfers the cargo into the recipient species.

The role of the host genotype in determining suitability as a host has been much better studied in *E. coli* than in any other Gram-negative bacteria (see Section 2.2.3). Many species have been shown to contain restriction enzymes that may degrade incoming DNA. These include the LT, SA, and SB systems of *Salmonella,* which are analogous to the Class I *E. coli hsd* system, and strains mutant in these are available. Many widely used Class II restriction enzymes come from Gram-negative bacteria, such as *Ava*I from the cyanobacterium *Anabaena variabilis*. Treatment of cells with ultraviolet light has been used in attempts to enhance transformation rates, and it is possible that this effect is mediated by alleviation of restriction systems. Recombination systems have also been identified in some Gram-negative bacteria, and there are strains

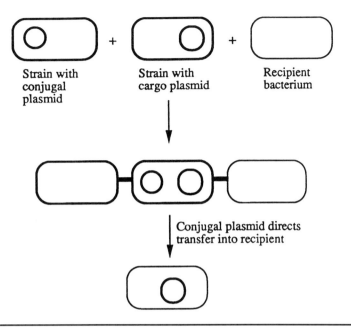

Figure 9.1 **Triparental mating to mobilize a cargo plasmid into a recipient.**

mutant in, for example, *recA* and *recBC* available for *Salmonella*. In some organisms, the recombination system may be indispensable – attempts to carry out gene disruption of a *recA* gene in some cyanobacteria have failed, suggesting that inactivation of the gene is lethal.

9. 2. 2 Vectors

The DNA used for transformation (or introduction by conjugation) could be in any of the following categories:

    a. Nonreplicating DNA. This can be linear material or circular material which, although perhaps able to replicate in *E. coli*, is not able to replicate in other hosts. It can therefore be stably maintained in the target species only by integration into another replicon, such as the bacterial chromosome, or another plasmid.

    b. A plasmid unique to the species under study. *E. coli* is, of course, not the only bacterial species to contain plasmids. However, it is more convenient if the plasmid used can replicate in *E. coli* as well as in the target species.

    c. A broad host-range plasmid. There are many broad host-range plasmids that are able to replicate in a number of different bacterial species. They can be classified into incompatibility groups on the basis that the presence in a cell of a plasmid of one group inhibits the replication of different plasmids from the same group. There are five separate incompatibility groups: C, N, P-1, Q, and W. Examples are given in Table 9.1. Members of the last three groups have been the most widely exploited for

TABLE 9.1 **Broad host-range plasmids of the P-1, Q, and W incompatibility groups.** Amp = ampicillin resistance, Kan = kanamycin resistance, Tet = tetracycline resistance, Str = streptomycin resistance, Sul = sulphonamide resistance.

PLASMID	GROUP	RESISTANCES	SIZE (kb)	TRANSMISSIBLE?
RK2	P-1	Amp, Kan, Tet	56.4	Self
RP301	P-1	Amp, Tet	54.7	Self
pRK2501	P-1	Kan, Tet	11.1	Nonmobilizable (derivative of RK2)
RSF101	Q	Str, Sul	8.9	Mobilizable
pKT254	Q	Str, Kan	12.8	Nonmobilizable
pGV1106	W	Sul, Kan	8.7	Mobilizable
pSa4	W	Cam, Str, Kan	9.4	Nonmobilizable

cloning purposes. Incompatibility group Q plasmids are smaller and of higher copy number than the others. They are unable to direct their own transfer (which reduces the risk of a modified plasmid's being accidentally released into the environment and becoming established), though they may be mobilizable by others. These factors favour their use, although suitable derivatives of the other groups are also available.

There are also many vectors that are artificially constructed hybrids between *E. coli* plasmids and plasmids specific to other species. They are therefore able to replicate and be selected in both species. They are called *shuttle vectors*, as they can be shuttled from one host to another, and they are very widely used. They are in effect functioning as artificially constructed broad host-range plasmids.

There are also cosmid vectors available with replication origins that can function in other Gram-negative bacteria in addition to *E. coli*. Likewise, there are expression vectors with powerful promoters from other Gram-negative species, such as the promoters from the genes for phycobiliproteins (proteins involved in light harvesting) from cyanobacteria, which can represent several percent of total cellular protein. In practice, many *E. coli* promoters will work in other Gram-negative species.

9. 3 GRAM-POSITIVE BACTERIA

9. 3. 1 Direct transformation

Gram-positive bacteria include a number of species, such as streptomycetes and actinomycetes, that carry out commercially important functions. They also include pathogens such as *Clostridium*. There is therefore considerable interest in the transformation of this group of bacteria, and one of the most widely studied species is *Bacillus subtilis*. A number of genera, such as *Bacillus*, *Streptomyces*, and *Streptococcus*, include species that exhibit natural compe-

tence. That is, they can take up exogenous DNA without the need for nonphysiological treatment, although the occurrence and efficiency of natural competence
can vary even within species. Competence is usually regulated, and is often determined by the excretion into the growth medium of extracellular, low-molecular-
weight proteins called *competence proteins*. Competence then develops as cell
density (and the concentration of competence proteins) in the medium increases.

The requirements for transforming DNA for *B. subtilis* are complex.
Plasmids that are capable of direct transformation into a host generally require
sequences that are also present on the host's chromosome, or sequences that are
also present on another plasmid already within the cell, or at least partial internal duplication of the plasmid sequence. It is probable that entry of the molecule
into the cell is associated with cutting and degradation of one strand.
Regeneration of a double-stranded molecule that can be replicated may then
depend on an inter- or intramolecular recombination event involving the incoming DNA. If recombination occurs between the incoming DNA and a sequence
in the host chromosome or an endogenous plasmid, the result is integration of
the DNA into that chromosome or plasmid. If the incoming DNA recombines
with itself in an intramolecular reaction, the result is recircularization. In addition, for some species the presence of a specific short nucleotide sequence
assists (or is essential for) plasmid uptake.

9. 3. 2   Protoplasts and other transformation procedures

The constraints on the types of plasmid that can be taken up by natural transformation can be relieved by the use of *protoplasts* (cells from which the walls
have been removed by treatment with lysozyme) from *B. subtilis* in the presence
of a suitable osmotic buffer (to stop cell lysis) and polyethylene glycol. Normal
cells are then regenerated from the protoplasts by transfer to a suitable medium.
The use of protoplasts somehow bypasses the stages that cause the linearization
and partial degradation of the incoming DNA. In some cases, it is possible to
use liposomes or even protoplasts of related species to transfer material.
Transformation of protoplasts is also the standard route for *Streptomyces* and
many other Gram-positive organisms. A disadvantage of protoplast transformation is that it may not be possible to use selection for markers (particularly
nutritional ones) in conjunction with the rich media used for regeneration of
normal cells from protoplasts. Furthermore, there are some species for which
neither protoplast nor natural transformation is possible.

Electroporation represents a third way of introducing DNA into a large
number of Gram-positive species, including *Bacillus,* and many that are otherwise refractory can be transformed by this means. Biolistic transformation
(described in Section 9.6.4) may also be used.

9. 3. 3   Hosts and vectors for B. subtilis

The considerations that apply for host and vector design for *B. subtilis* are the
same as those for *E. coli* and other Gram-negative bacteria. In addition to host
nutritional markers, such as *trpC2, leuB6,* and *metB10* (blocking tryptophan,
leucine, and methionine biosynthesis respectively in *B. subtilis*), there are mutations available – such as *recE4* – that lead to reductions in recombination and
consequent plasmid instability, as well as mutations that reduce endogenous
restriction enzyme activity.

TABLE 9.2 Plasmids for genetic manipulation of B. subtilis and other Gram-positive species.
Ery = erythromycin resistance, Tet = tetracycline resistance, Cam = chloramphenicol resistance, Kan = kanamycin resistance, Trp = tryptophan biosynthesis.

PLASMID	SOURCE	MARKERS	SIZE (kb)
pIM13	*B. subtilis*	Ery	2.3
pBC16	*B. cereus*	Tet	4.5
pC194	*S. aureus*	Cam	2.9
pE194	*S. aureus*	Ery	3.7
pUB110	*S. aureus*	Kan	4.5
pBD64	pC194, pUB110	Cam, Kan	4.7
pLS103	*B. pumilis trp* gene, pUB110	Trp, Kan	8.1
pHV33	pC194, pBR322	Cam, Amp, Tet	7.3

Stable retention of incoming DNA is possible by its integration into the chromosome, as well as by its maintenance as a plasmid, but integration into the chromosome makes any subsequent re-isolation of the incoming DNA very difficult, so it is better to use a plasmid where possible. Many plasmid vectors exploited for manipulation of *B. subtilis* are based on plasmids isolated from *Staphylococcus aureus* as well as *Bacillus* species. A number of plasmids are listed in Table 9.2, including vectors conferring multiple drug resistance phenotypes generated by recombining the plasmids *in vitro*. Insertion of selectable *E. coli* plasmids into the *Bacillus* or *S. aureus* plasmids generates shuttle vectors such as pHV33 (also shown in Table 9.2). There are also *B. subtilis* bacteriophage vectors available, which can be used in much the same way as lambda derivatives and *E. coli*, but the technology is less developed.

9. 3. 4 Expression in B. subtilis

One of the most attractive reasons for using *B. subtilis* as a cloning host is that it can be used quite effectively for overexpression and for secretion directly into the culture medium (whereas secretion from *E. coli* cells is generally into the periplasmic space and no further). A potential problem with this is that *B. subtilis* also secretes a number of proteases into its culture medium. However, strains that are deficient in a number of these proteases have been constructed, allowing in principle an enhancement of the stability of secreted proteins. Several expression systems are available. One controllable system is based on the use of the *E. coli lac* repressor. Modification of the *lacI* gene by attachment of a *B. subtilis* promoter and ribosome binding site allows the production of LacI in *B. subtilis*. If the *E. coli lac* operator is then joined to a suitable promoter, LacI-mediated control of that promoter (using IPTG) becomes possible. One such promoter that has been successfully fused to the *lac* operator is the

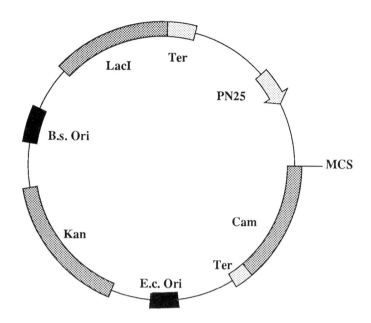

Figure 9.2 **Plasmid pREP9 (7.3 kb), an example of a B. *subtilis* expression vector.** Sequences inserted into the multiple cloning site (MCS) are expressed from the *lac* operator–P_{N25} promoter (PN25). The plasmid can function as a shuttle vector, with origins for replication in *E. coli* (E.c.) or *Bacillus subtilis* (B.s.).

P_{N25} promoter from the *E. coli* bacteriophage T5, which is functional in *B. subtilis*, but homologous promoters can also be used – for example, from the *Bacillus* phage SPO1. The modified *lacI* gene and the *lac*-P_{N25} promoter can be included in the same plasmid, as shown in Figure 9.2, or they can be carried on different ones. The plasmid shown in Figure 9.2, pREP9, has a ribosome binding site and a multiple cloning site for DNA insertion, a chloramphenicol acetyltransferase reporter gene, a transcription terminator, a kanamycin resistance selectable marker, and Gram-negative and Gram-positive origins of replication (allowing use as a shuttle vector). A potential problem with this system is that at different growth stages (e.g., during sporulation) of *B. subtilis*, different promoters become active. Under these circumstances, expression of the modified *lacI* and perhaps also the *lac*-P_{N25} promoters may be considerably reduced.

Secretion from *B. subtilis* is usually directed by production of a fusion polypeptide with part of one of the proteins that are normally secreted by *Bacillus* species, such as alpha-amylase, alkaline protease (subtilisin), neutral protease, and levansucrase. Although several of these come from different species (for example, alpha-amylase and alkaline protease are produced by *B. amyloliquefaciens*), the amino-termini of these proteins function satisfactorily in *B. subtilis* as leader peptides.

9. 3. 5 Other Gram-positive bacteria

Some of the plasmids available for *Bacillus subtilis* can be used in other bacteria. Endogenous plasmids can also be used – on their own, or for the construction of shuttle vectors. For example, the plasmid pIJ61, derived ultimately from *Streptomyces coelicolor*, can be used in several *Streptomyces* species and con-

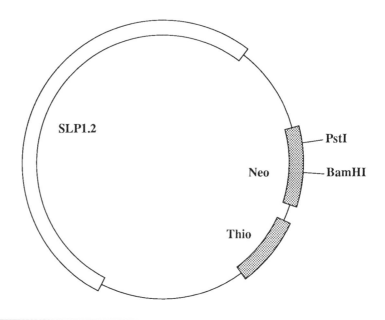

Figure 9.3 Streptomyces vector pIJ61 (15.7 kb). The region marked SLP1.2 derived from *S. coelicolor*, where it existed as an integrated plasmid. The vector contains genes for resistance to neomycin (Neo) and thiostrepton (Thio) for use as selectable markers.

tains genes for resistance to neomycin and thiostrepton as selectable markers (Figure 9.3). The plasmid pAL5000 from *Mycobacterium fortuitum* has been used for the construction of shuttle vectors for mycobacteria. There are also vectors based on phages, such as the actinophage PhiC31 and the temperate mycobacteriophage L5. Expression systems are available for some species.

9. 4   FUNGI

The fungi are an extremely diverse group of organisms. The best studied is the ascomycete fungus *Saccharomyces cerevisiae* ("yeast"), so we will concentrate on that. However, vectors and transformation systems have been developed for a number of other fungi, including species that are of particular interest as pathogens for plants and animals, so we will look briefly at some of those as well. In this section, we will deal just with the nuclear genome. Manipulation of the yeast mitochondrial genome is discussed later, in Section 9.7.2.

9. 4. 1   Transformation systems

There are a number of ways available for introducing exogenous DNA into *S. cerevisiae*. One of the easiest is probably simply treatment of the cells with lithium acetate and polyethylene glycol, together with the transforming DNA and extra nonspecific "carrier" DNA (for example, from calf thymus) to increase the total amount of DNA present. Although this method is relatively straightforward, the efficiency of transfer can be rather low, approximately 10^3 colonies per microgram of plasmid, although higher frequencies have been claimed and may represent differences between strains.

A second – and often more efficient – approach to introducing exogenous DNA into *S. cerevisiae* is the transformation of spheroplasts, which are obtained by digestion of the cell wall with appropriate enzymes, in the presence of a suitable osmotic buffer to prevent lysis. The spheroplasts are exposed to the transforming DNA, in the presence of polyethylene glycol and calcium chloride. The next step is to regenerate intact cells from spheroplasts. This is achieved by immobilizing the spheroplasts in a suitable agar that is osmotically buffered. Surrounding the spheroplasts with a solid medium allows the retention of cell wall material around the cell during the earliest and most sensitive stages of cell wall regeneration.

A third method for introduction of DNA into *S. cerevisiae* is electroporation, which we have already encountered in bacterial transformation (see Section 2.2.2). It is reported that this method can give tenfold higher efficiency than spheroplast transformation, although the actual figure seems to vary quite widely. As with other electroporation systems, the cells are simply subjected to an electric field pulse. There is no need to make spheroplasts for this treatment. Other methods include particle bombardment (see Section 9.6.4) and cell damage by agitation with glass beads. Transmission of DNA from *E. coli* by conjugation has also been reported; the *E. coli* cells must contain a plasmid that can replicate both in *E. coli* and in yeast (i.e., a shuttle vector) and a second plasmid, which mobilizes the first.

9. 4. 2 Markers

One of the most commonly used selectable markers is the *URA3* gene. This encodes orotidine-5'-phosphate decarboxylase, an enzyme of uracil biosynthesis. Acquisition of a functional *URA3* gene by cells that were previously mutant at this locus allows them to grow in the absence of exogenous uracil. Examples of other frequently used selectable markers that can be selected in a similar way are given in Table 9.3. *TUN*[R] confers resistance to the antibiotic tunicamycin, an inhibitor of glycosylation. *Lack of SUP4* (an ochre chain termination suppressor) can be selected in suitable host backgrounds. One such host has an

Table 9.3 Selectable markers for use in *S. cerevisiae*

MARKER	FUNCTION
URA3	orotidine-5'-phosphate decarboxylase (in *de novo* synthesis of pyrimidines)
LEU2	ß-isopropylmalate dehydrogenase (in leucine biosynthesis)
HIS3	imidazole glycerol phosphate dehydratase (in histidine biosynthesis)
TRP1	N-(5'-phosphoribosyl)anthranilate isomerase (in tryptophan biosynthesis)
TUN[R]	UDP-N-acetylglucosamine-1-P transferase (in glycosylation; confers tunicamycin resistance)
SUP4	tyrosine-tRNA (ochre suppressor)

ochre chain termination mutation in the *CAN1* gene. The wild-type gene encodes a permease that causes uptake of the toxic arginine analogue canavanine and, consequently, causes cell death in the presence of canavanine. So *can1* mutant cells are resistant to canavanine, as they are unable to take it up. However, the chain termination suppressor *SUP4* causes the production of functional permease in the *can1* background (because it suppresses the *can1* mutation) and therefore causes the death of *can1* cells in the presence of canavanine. Loss of *SUP4* abolishes canavanine uptake and causes canavanine resistance, which can readily be selected. Cells containing *SUP4* can also be identified by the use of hosts with a chain termination mutation in the *ADE2* gene for phosphoribosyl amino-imidazole carboxylase, a component of the arginine biosynthesis pathway. The mutation causes the cells to accumulate a red pigment, whereas colonies are the usual colour if they are wild type or if the ochre mutation is suppressed by *SUP4*. Cells that have lost *SUP4* therefore acquire the red pigment and are visibly distinguishable from the others.

9. 4. 3 Vectors

The plasmid vectors used commonly in yeast can be divided into two categories: Yeast Centromeric plasmid (YCp) and Yeast Episomal plasmid (YEp) vectors. An example of a YCp plasmid is given in Figure 9.4. It contains prokaryotic ampicillin and tetracycline resistance genes and an origin of replication for *E. coli*, all in a region of the plasmid derived from pBR322. These will allow it to function as a shuttle vector, and sequences can be cloned into the ampicillin or tetracycline resistance genes. Many of the yeast vectors are based on

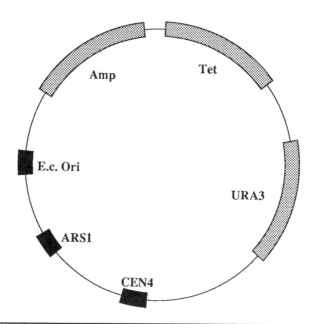

Figure 9.4 **Yeast centromeric plasmid YCp50 (7.9 kb).** The presence of a suitable origin (E.c. Ori) and selectable markers (Amp and Tet) allows it to be used as a shuttle vector in *E. coli*. The vector contains a yeast selectable marker (URA3), a centromeric sequence (CEN4), and an autonomously replicating sequence (ARS1).

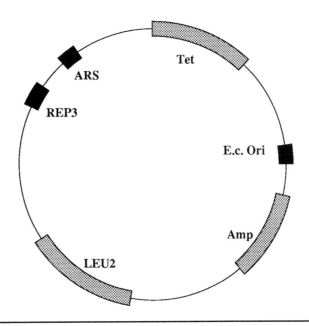

Figure 9.5 Yeast episomal plasmid YEp13 (10.8 kb). The presence of a suitable origin (E.c. Ori) and selectable markers (Amp and Tet) allows it to be used as a shuttle vector in *E. coli*. The vector contains a yeast selectable marker (LEU2), a partitioning sequence (REP3), and an autonomously replicating sequence (ARS) derived from the 2μ plasmid.

pBR322 in this way, but other plasmids have also been used, including pUC and Bluescript species (Sections 2.3.2 and 3.2.4). There are also a selectable marker and an origin of replication for yeast, ARS1. (ARS, or autonomously replicating sequences, are those that confer on a plasmid the ability to replicate without integration into another replicon. There are several available from yeast.) The distinguishing feature of YCp plasmids is the presence of a chromosomal centromeric sequence, *CEN4* in this example. The presence of a centromeric sequence allows the plasmid to be partitioned by the spindle apparatus of the cell, in the same way that the endogenous chromosomes are partitioned. Although this also results in a reduction of the copy number per cell, it confers a much greater stability during cell division, allowing the plasmid to be maintained in the absence of selection.

An example of a YEp vector is shown in Figure 9.5. Most of the features are similar to those of YCp plasmids, except for the absence of the centromeric sequence and its replacement with a different origin of replication. This comes from a naturally occurring episomal plasmid from yeast, called the 2μ circle. As well as the origin of replication, there is a naturally occurring *cis*-acting sequence, *REP3*, which is the site of action for two proteins that help in the partitioning of the plasmid during cell division. This gives the YEp vectors a mitotic stability similar to that of the YCp vectors, but with a somewhat higher copy number. It may be possible to increase copy number further by use of a selectable marker (e.g., some alleles of *LEU2*) that complements only poorly. This gives a selective advantage to cells with a higher plasmid copy number.

There are more sophisticated versions of these classes of vectors, with further modifications. These include the presence of filamentous phage origins, for generation of single-stranded DNA; and the *lacZ* system, for detecting the presence of inserts when the vectors are used in *E. coli*.

Stable transformation is of course also possible by integration of the incoming DNA into the chromosome using homologous recombination. This will clearly make recovery of the transforming DNA much more difficult than when a plasmid is used. Integration is the basis of gene disruption (see Section 7.7.1).

9. 4. 4 Expression systems

There are several controllable promoters available for expression in yeast, including those for two of the genes of galactose metabolism, *GAL1* and *GAL10,* encoding galactokinase and UDP-galactose-4-epimerase (Figure 9.6). When wild-type control proteins are present, transcription of *GAL1* and *GAL10* is increased greatly in the presence of galactose. In the presence of glucose, transcription is tightly repressed. These promoters, together with their upstream controlling sequences, can be used either in expression vectors or as cassettes for insertion into other constructs. Other promoters that can be tightly controlled and are used for expression purposes include those from *PGK* (3-phosphoglycerate kinase), *ADH1* (alcohol dehydrogenase I), and *PHO5,* a secreted acid phosphatase. The *PGK* and *ADH1* promoters are active in media containing glucose and can be repressed by growth on nonfermentable carbon sources, such as acetate. *PHO5* is active when the medium lacks inorganic phosphate (presumably to help in phosphate scavenging), and is very strongly repressed in the presence of inorganic phosphate. These promoters can be used to direct the synthesis of either unmodified proteins or fusion proteins; the latter can incorporate either the corresponding products of *GAL10, PGK,* and so forth, or other sequences, such as LacZ or TrpE from *E. coli*. There are also constitutive promoters available; for example, from the gene for glyceraldehyde-3-phosphate dehydrogenase. An advantage with using yeast rather than prokaryotic cells for expression of eukaryotic proteins is that posttranslational modifications of the proteins – such as glycosylation, phosphorylation, and acylation – are unlikely

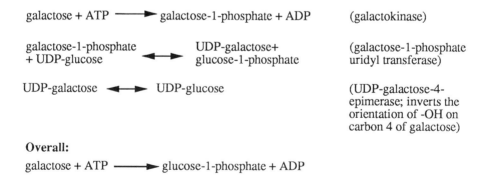

Overall:

galactose + ATP ⟶ glucose-1-phosphate + ADP

Figure 9.6 **Metabolism of galactose.** The glucose-1-phosphate can be converted to glucose-6-phosphate through glucose-1,6-*bis*-phosphate and then metabolized by glycolysis or other standard routes.

to take place in prokaryotic systems but may well do so in yeast. Even in yeast, these modifications may not take place reliably, and it may be necessary to use expression in insect or mammalian cells (see Sections 9.8.1 and 9.9.1).

9. 4. 5 Secretion systems

Secretion of overexpressed proteins by fusion to a secretion signal may be useful because it assists purification and allows the proteins produced to be only minimally exposed to most of the yeast proteases. In addition, it may help to bring about correct glycosylation and may also enhance protein folding. A number of secretion signals, from both yeast and other organisms, can be used. The most commonly used are probably those for the mating pheromone alpha-peptide and for invertase (product of the *SUC2* gene). The mating pheromone is a 13-residue peptide, secreted from cells of alpha mating type, that acts on a receptor on a-type cells. Invertase is secreted in order to bring about the breakdown of extracellular sucrose to glucose and fructose.

9. 4. 6 Yeast artificial chromosomes (YACs)

Yeast artificial chromosomes are sophisticated vectors that can be used for propagating large stretches (in the megabase size-range) of DNA. This is very useful, because it reduces the number of recombinants needed to cover the entire genome of an organism. The aim is to synthesize an artificial chromosome that can be maintained in yeast, but which is composed mostly of foreign DNA. An example is shown in Figure 9.7, together with a representative cloning strategy. The vector contains *HIS3, URA3, TRP1,* and *SUP4,* described in Section 9.4.2. *CEN4* is a centromeric sequence, and *TEL* is a telomeric sequence derived from the ends of ribosomal RNA-encoding molecules from the macronucleus of *Tetrahymena.* In addition, there are a yeast origin of replication, a prokaryotic origin of replication, and an ampicillin resistance gene. The latter two features allow YAC DNA to be prepared from *E. coli* prior to the cloning. The whole molecule is just over 10 kb.

The YAC DNA is digested, in this case, with *Bam*HI and *Sma*I; this generates three fragments, two of which contain *TEL* sequences and are the ones we will need. (The third has the *HIS3* gene.) Subsequent religation of the fragments can be prevented by treatment with phosphatase. The DNA is then mixed with the insert material – which has been prepared in a way that leaves blunt ends – and ligated, and the ligation products are transformed into yeast by the means already described in this chapter (Section 9.4.1). There they can function as *bona fide* chromosomes possessing a centromere, an origin of replication, and telomeres. Transformed cells can be selected by the presence of the *URA3* and *TRP1* genes. The presence of both of these indicates that both arms of the YAC have been acquired. Screening for the inactivation of *SUP4* allows putative recombinants to be identified.

There are several modifications to this basic YAC design. One is the incorporation of an extra prokaryotic origin and prokaryotic selectable marker, so that there is one of each on each arm. That assists in the recovery of at least parts of individual recombinant YACs using *E. coli*. The YAC DNA is isolated from yeast, digested, self-ligated, and used to transform *E. coli*. Cells containing either the left arm or the right arm can then be selected (Figure 9.8). Bacteriophage promoters (T7, etc.) can also be included to allow the synthesis of RNA transcripts *in vitro*.

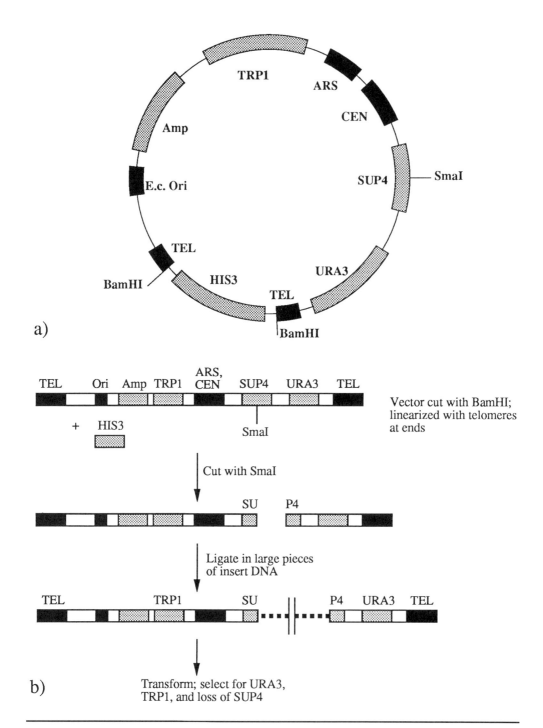

Figure 9.7 YAC cloning. Panel **(a)** shows a representative YAC, pYAC2; panel **(b)** shows a typical cloning strategy. Note the telomeres (TEL) that constitute the ends of the linear recombinant molecule, as shown in panel **(b)**. Other sequences are as described in the text. The inserted DNA is indicated by the broken dashed line.

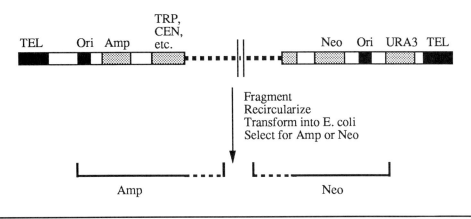

Figure 9.8 **YAC cloning and recovery in *E. coli.*** Note the presence of a prokaryotic origin and drug resistance gene (ampicillin or neomycin resistance) in each arm, allowing recovery of each arm and adjacent inserted sequence.

9. 4. 7 Other fungi

Another unicellular fungus that is widely studied is the fission yeast *Schizosaccharomyces pombe.* As its name implies, this reproduces by fission, in contrast to *Saccharomyces cerevisiae,* which reproduces by budding. Similar principles apply with *Schizosaccharomyces pombe* as with *Saccharomyces cerevisiae*, although integration of DNA into the chromosome is less efficient, reflecting a lower frequency of homologous recombination under standard conditions in *Schizosaccharomyces pombe.* As with *Saccharomyces cerevisiae,* the plasmids used generally contain a prokaryotic origin of replication and selectable marker, and a yeast origin and marker. In fact, the pBR322 origin itself is functional inside *S. pombe*, although plasmids based on this give a rather low transformation frequency. The frequency can be improved by incorporation of a yeast origin of replication. The *Saccharomyces cerevisiae* 2μm origin can be used, although the resulting plasmids are rather unstable. At least one *Schizosaccharomyces pombe* autonomously replicating sequence (*ars*) has also been used; the stability of these plasmids is rather variable. Perhaps surprisingly, although the transformation efficiency is increased by incorporation of a yeast replication origin, the resulting copy number is decreased.

Commonly used selectable markers from *Schizosaccharomyces pombe* are *ura4+* and *sup3-5*. The former complements mutations in the *ura4* gene, for orotidine-5'-phosphate decarboxylase (an enzyme of pyrimidine biosynthesis). The *sup3-5* allele suppresses an *ade* mutation, as with *Saccharomyces cerevisiae,* allowing the colour selection described previously (Section 9.4.2). It is also possible to use the markers *LEU2* and *URA3* from *Saccharomyces cerevisiae,* complementing the *Schizosaccharomyces pombe* mutations *leu1⁻* and *ura4⁻*, although they are less reliable.

Expression vectors are also available, with three promoters being commonly used. These promoters are derived from the *adh* gene for alcohol dehydrogenase, which is constitutive; the *fbp* gene for fructose *bis*-phosphatase, tightly repressed in the presence of glucose; and the *nmt* gene, which is presumed to be involved in thiamine biosynthesis, since it is not transcribed in the presence of thiamine (i.e., there is **no** **m**essage from it in **t**hiamine).

Other yeasts may have more efficient secretion systems than *Saccharomyces* and *Schizosaccharomyces; Kluyveromyces lactis* is of interest in this respect. There are integration vectors available, and also vectors for extrachromosomal replication using chromosomal ARS sequences or origins from naturally occurring *Kluyveromyces* plasmids. Secretion can be directed by fusion to suitable sequences from a secreted toxin that kills other cells.

Filamentous fungi, such as *Aspergillus nidulans* (and other *Aspergillus* species), *Neurospora crassa,* and *Penicillium chrysogenum,* are also of considerable interest. Transformation can be carried out with protoplasts made from spores or hyphae, by digestion of the cell wall with suitable enzymes. DNA is added in the presence of calcium ions and polyethylene glycol. The latter apparently causes protoplast fusion, and DNA is taken up at the same time. Electroporation can also be used. The protoplasts are then regenerated. Ensuring stable maintenance of extrachromosomal molecules is difficult, because of the filamentous nature of the fungi. As a result of this filamentous habit, cells that have lost a selectable marker can be maintained by those cells in the filament that have retained it. Using a system that results in integration of incoming DNA may therefore be more convenient. Integration can occur quite easily by both heterologous and homologous recombination. Several selectable markers are available, and common examples are given in Table 9.4. Some of these, such as *argB,* require the availability of the appropriately mutant strain as a recipient. Controlled expression can be directed conveniently from the *alcA* promoter, for alcohol dehydrogenase, in response to the carbon substrate.

There is also a lot of interest in the transformation of pathogenic fungi of both plants and animals. Frequently, transformation can be achieved by treatment of protoplasts with the DNA in the presence of polyethylene glycol and cal-

TABLE 9.4 Selectable markers for use in filamentous fungi

MARKER	SOURCE	PRODUCT	PHENOTYPE
argB	*Aspergillus nidulans*	ornithine transcarbamoylase	ability to synthesize arginine
hph	*E. coli*	hygromycin phosphotransferase	hygromycin resistance (phosphorylates it)
ble	*Streptoalloteichus hindustanus*	bleomycin-binding protein	bleomycin resistance (binds to it and inhibits its DNA-damaging activity)
benA	*Aspergillus nidulans*	beta-tubulin	resistance to fungicide benomyl
amdS	*Aspergillus nidulans*	acetamidase	growth on acetamide as sole carbon or nitrogen source

cium chloride. A number of selectable markers derived from one fungus can be used in others. For example, the *argB⁺* gene from *Aspergillus nidulans* has been used as a selectable marker in a suitably mutant strain of *Magnaporthe grisea,* the causative agent of rice blast disease. Similarly, the *niaD⁺* (nitrate reductase) gene of *Aspergillus nidulans* can be used in a *niaD⁻* strain of *Fusarium oxysporum,* another plant pathogen. Alternatively, bacterial genes attached to suitable expression sequences can be used. The *E. coli* hygromycin B phosphotransferase gene *hph,* attached to suitable fungal expression signals, is widely used to confer resistance to the antibiotic. This marker has the advantage of eliminating the need for development of suitable mutant recipient strains. Heterologous fungal promoters can be used for expression of *hph.* For example, the *Ustilago maydis hsp70* heat shock gene promoter has been used to drive expression in fungi belonging to the important pathogenic genus *Phytophthora,* and *Aspergillus nidulans* signals have been used for *Trichoderma,* a genus including a number of important biological control agents.

The fate of the incoming DNA depends upon whether or not a suitable replication origin is present. ARS elements have been isolated, such as UARS1 from *Ustilago maydis,* which allow maintenance as a plasmid. Some ARS elements may function in heterologous species. For example, the origin of the *Saccharomyces cerevisiae* 2µ plasmid can support replication in a number of other species. Alternatively, DNA may be integrated into host chromosomes by homologous or nonhomologous recombination.

9. 5 CHLAMYDOMONAS

The unicellular green alga *Chlamydomonas* has been used for many purposes as a model plant system (despite the fact that it is clearly a rather different organism from multicellular land plants). The earliest experiments on nuclear transformation used protoplasts. These can be generated by treatment of intact cells with *autolysin,* a cell-wall digesting activity that is produced by gamete cells immediately prior to mating. More conveniently, mutants – such as the *cw-15* strain – exist that lack cell walls and hence form a "natural" protoplast. It has been reported that protoplasts could be transformed by treatment with DNA in the presence of poly-L-ornithine and polyethylene glycol or zinc sulphate, but many of these experiments gave very low and variable transformation rates. Particle bombardment (see Section 9.6.4), which does not require the absence of a cell wall, was found to give more efficient and reliable transformation. Subsequently it has been found that simple, rapid mixing of protoplasts with the DNA in the presence of glass beads gives even higher transformation frequencies. Electroporation can also be used.

Selectable markers include the following:

a. the yeast *ARG4* gene, encoding the enzyme argininosuccinate lyase (an enzyme of arginine biosynthesis, converting argininosuccinate to arginine and fumarate), which can be used to complement *Chlamydomonas arg7* mutations

b. a bacterial neomycin phosphotransferase gene under the control of a suitable promoter (actually the early promoter from the mammalian virus SV40), conferring resistance to the aminoglycoside antibiotics G418 and kanamycin

c. the *Chlamydomonas* nitrate reductase *NIT1* gene, allowing *nit1* mutant cells to grow in the presence of nitrate as the sole nitrogen source

d. the *OEE1* gene, a component of Photosystem II, allowing mutant cells lacking that polypeptide (the FuD44 strain) to grow photoautotrophically

Other selectable markers include genes for other enzymes of nitrogen metabolism, and genes for components of the flagellum. If one marker is selected for, it is often found that other sequences, unlinked and unselected, have also been acquired. This phenomenon is called *cotransformation*. Although ARS sequences have been obtained from *Chlamydomonas*, most experiments simply use integration of DNA into the chromosome, which gives efficient transformation. Another very important application of *Chlamydomonas* transformation is the manipulation of the chloroplast rather than the nucleus; this is described in Section 9.7.1

9. 6 VASCULAR PLANTS

A wide range of methods have been used for the transformation of plant cells. Different methods tend to use different vectors, so we will consider vector systems at the same time as transformation systems. The main methods that we will consider are *Agrobacterium*-mediated transfer, direct transfer into protoplasts, particle-gun (biolistic) transformation, and viral transformation.

9. 6. 1 *Agrobacterium*-mediated transfer

One of the most widely used approaches for the introduction of DNA into plant cells exploits the natural DNA-transferring properties of a soil-inhabiting bacterium, *Agrobacterium tumefaciens*. A related species, *Agrobacterium rhizogenes,* can also be used. The two species cause the diseases crown gall and hairy root, respectively, on plants. The two species belong to the Rhizobiaceae, which include other important genera, such as *Rhizobium.* Both lead to disturbance of normal plant growth, causing in one case a gall and in the other, abnormal roots. Their ability to do so depends on the presence of large plasmids, in excess of 100 kb, which are referred to as the "Tumour-inducing" (or Ti) and "Root-inducing" (or Ri) plasmids respectively. We will concentrate on the Ti plasmids; the Ri plasmids are quite similar.

A simplified diagram of a Ti plasmid is shown in Figure 9.9. Most important is a region referred to as the T-DNA ("Transferred DNA"), which is transferred from an infecting *Agrobacterium* cell into the nucleus of the plant cell, where it is integrated into the plant genome. Transfer of the T-DNA depends on a set of genes called *vir* if they are on the Ti plasmid, or *chv* if they are on the chromosome. They are induced in response to various compounds in exudates from wounded plants; these compounds include acetosyringone; alpha-hydroxy-acetosyringone; and precursors of lignin, such as coniferyl alcohol. The T-DNA itself is flanked by repeated sequences of around 25 base pairs, called *border repeats* (or left and right borders). The T-DNA contains a group of genes referred to as the *onc* genes, as they are responsible for the T-DNA's oncogenicity (or tumour-inducing potential). They include genes for the synthesis of an auxin and a cytokinin, which are plant growth regulators that cause the disturbance of cell growth. In addition, the T-DNA contains genes for enzymes

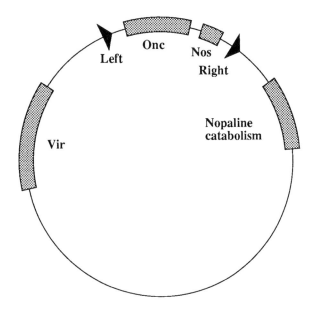

Figure 9.9 Simplified diagram of a Ti plasmid.. Arrowheads indicate the left and right borders of the region transferred (the T-DNA). Onc genes are responsible for growth transformation, nos for nopaline synthase, and vir for transfer of the T-DNA into a target cell.

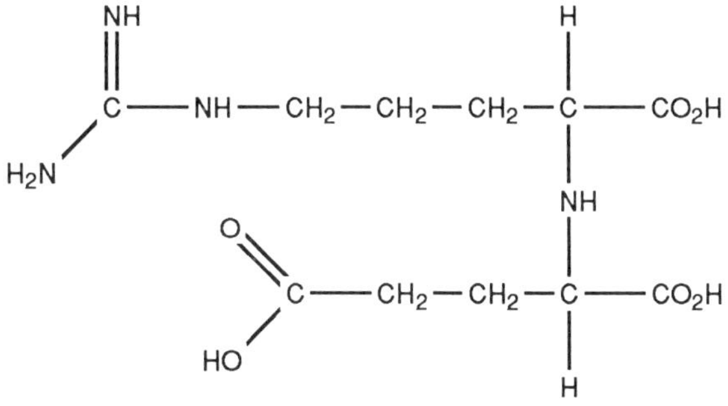

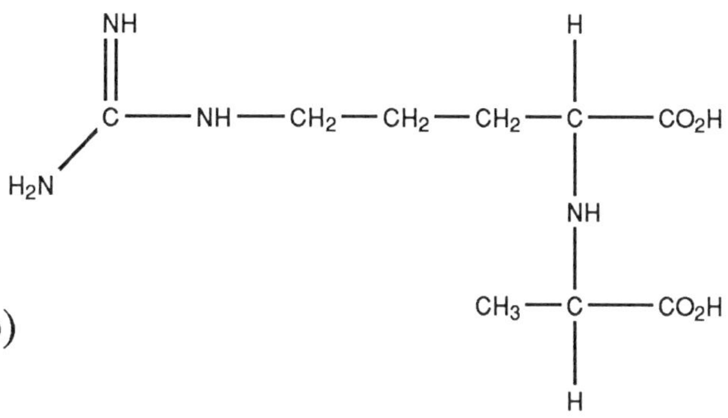

Figure 9.10 Examples of opines: nopaline (a) and octopine (b).

that produce unusual amino acid conjugates, such as nopaline and octopine (Figure 9.10), collectively called opines. Therefore, plant cells that have had T-DNA incorporated will grow in an apparently uncontrolled way and will synthesize opines. The opines are excreted by the plant cells – which are unable to utilize them themselves – and are utilized instead by *Agrobacterium* cells near the site of infection, whose Ti plasmids also contain genes for opine breakdown. *Agrobacterium* therefore has a very sophisticated mechanism for subverting the normal cell function.

The basic principle of using *Agrobacterium* as a tool for plant genetic manipulation is to insert foreign DNA into the T-DNA of a bacterial cell and rely on the bacterium to transfer the DNA into the plant. As long as the necessary proteins are provided by the bacterium, any sequences flanked by the T-DNA border repeats can be transferred into the recipient plant cell genome. Unfortunately, the Ti plasmids are rather too large to manipulate directly, but the problem can be circumvented in different ways.

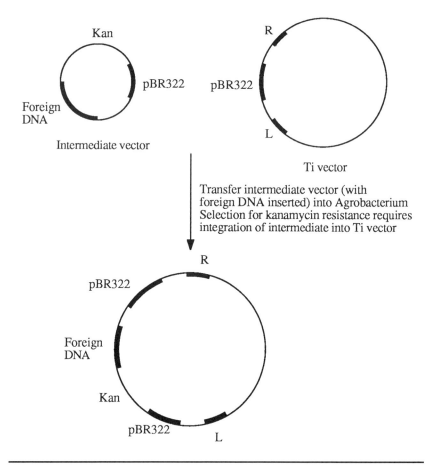

*Figure 9.11 **Agrobacterium** cointegrative vector system.* L and R indicate the left and right borders in the Ti vector. The system relies on homologous recombination across pBR322 sequences common to both the intermediate vector and the Ti vector to integrate the former into the latter.

COINTEGRATIVE SYSTEMS. A cointegrative vector system is summarized in Figure 9.11. Its two main components are a Ti plasmid that has been modified by the replacement of much of the material between the border repeats (including the *onc* sequences) by pBR322; and an intermediate vector, which is a modified pBR322 containing an extra marker, such as kanamycin resistance. The gene to be introduced into the target plant is first cloned into the intermediate vector, and this construct is then introduced into *Agrobacterium* containing the Ti vector. The pBR322-based plasmid cannot replicate efficiently inside *Agrobacterium*, so selection for kanamycin resistance identifies those *Agrobacterium* cells where the pBR322-based intermediate plasmid (which therefore contains the gene to be introduced into the target plant) has been integrated by homologous recombination into the Ti plasmid. Because the recombination is homologous, it will take place across the pBR322 sequences and therefore result in integration between the border repeats. *Agrobacterium* containing this modified Ti plasmid can then be used for plant transformation as described in "Transfer into plant cells" (later in Section 9.6.1).

BINARY SYSTEMS. The need for cointegration of the plasmids can be circumvented by use of a binary vector, such as pBin19, shown in Figure 9.12. This is a small plasmid containing a pair of left and right borders. Within the borders are the *lacZ* region, to assist insertion and detection of DNA, and a neomycin phosphotransferase gene, modified for expression in plants by addition of nopaline synthase expression sequences. Outside the left and right borders, there are a kanamycin resistance gene that will function in prokaryotes, and a broad host-

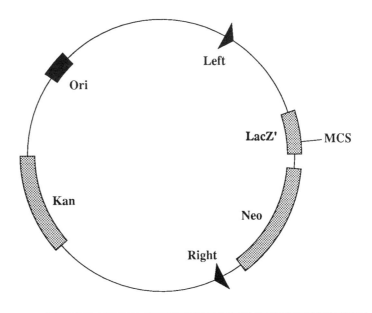

Figure 9.12 **Plasmid pBin19 (10.0 kb).** There are a broad host-range origin of replication (Ori) and kanamycin resistance gene (Kan) for propagation of the plasmid in prokaryotic hosts; the neomycin resistance gene (Neo) is for selection in plants. There is a multiple cloning site (MCS) in the *lac* minigene (LacZ').

range origin (Section 9.2.2) derived from the plasmid pRK252. The proteins that catalyse transfer of the T-DNA into the host plant do not have to be *cis*-encoded (i.e., do not have to be encoded by the same molecule). Therefore, if the binary vector is introduced into *Agrobacterium* that already contains a resident Ti plasmid, the resident plasmid can provide all the functions needed for transfer into a plant nucleus of the DNA between the borders of the binary vector. There are also more sophisticated binary vectors – for example, pROK1 – that have plant promoters incorporated to drive expression. Others have *cos* sites to allow packaging into lambda phage heads.

When the correct sequences have been incorporated into a vector (whether binary or cointegrative), it must then be transferred to an *Agrobacterium* strain carrying an appropriate Ti plasmid. This is usually done either by electroporation with naked DNA or by a triparental mating involving the *Agrobacterium* strain, an *E. coli* strain containing the vector to be transferred, and an *E. coli* strain with a plasmid capable of mobilizing the binary or intermediate vector into *Agrobacterium*.

TRANSFER INTO PLANT CELLS. Once the binary vector or the cointegrative vector has been introduced into a suitable *Agrobacterium* strain (and cointegration has occurred), the next stage is to arrange for the *Agrobacterium* to infect plant cells. Various methods exist, including inoculation of intact plants with *Agrobacterium* cultures by injection, but the most widely used is to incubate discs cut from leaves of the target plant with an *Agrobacterium* culture. The bacterium will attack cells round the edge of the wounded leaf disc and transfer its T-DNA into them. The leaf discs are then transferred to a suitable medium to select for transformation. The neomycin phosphotransferase gene mentioned earlier is widely used, conferring resistance to aminoglycoside antibiotics, such as neomycin, kanamycin, and G418. On a suitable selective medium, shoots form around the edges of the treated leaf discs. The shoots can then be regenerated into intact plants. (The medium also contains another antibiotic, to kill remaining *Agrobacterium* cells.) The resulting plants can have several copies of the incoming DNA integrated at more or less random sites, sometimes with rearrangements, so detailed analysis of the transformed plants is necessary – but the plant tissue culture side of things can often be the most technically difficult part of the operation.

9. 6. 2 Protoplast transformation

Direct transformation of protoplasts without using *Agrobacterium* is possible and might seem a much simpler means of going about plant transformation. Uptake of naked DNA can be brought about by treatment with polyethylene glycol, or by electroporation. DNA is integrated into the recipient genome, and in some cases this appears to be brought about by homologous recombination. Selection for transformants can be done using the same selectable markers as are used in *Agrobacterium* transformation. However, the most difficult aspect of this approach is the regeneration of intact plants from protoplasts. Although regeneration is possible for many plants (unlike most other eukaryotes), for many agriculturally important plants it is very difficult. For these plants, *Agrobacterium*-mediated transformation and regeneration may well be equally difficult, though – so there is rarely an easy solution.

9. 6. 3 Transient expression

For some experiments, it may not be necessary to regenerate intact plants. For example, many studies on the regulatory elements necessary for the expression of particular genes have been carried out by introducing the elements (or modifications of them) into protoplasts and then monitoring expression. Because the transformation is not stable, these experiments are called *transient expression* systems (although if things are working well, expression can be followed for days). It should always be borne in mind, when interpreting the results of these experiments, that expression in protoplasts can be rather different from expression in the intact tissue, but for many situations the results appear quite reliable. Another approach to transient expression involves the use of the particle gun (see Section 9.6.4) to introduce sequences into intact tissues prior to monitoring expression.

9. 6. 4 Biolistic transformation: the particle gun

One of the less subtle (but extremely effective) methods for introducing DNA into plant cells is to coat it onto the surface of tiny particles of material such as tungsten or gold, and fire them into the target cells. This can be done using a particle gun, powered by an explosive charge (as shown in Figure 9.13) or compressed gas. The explosion forces forward a macroprojectile, which in turn forces forward the DNA-coated microprojectiles. The macroprojectile is stopped by a pierced plate, which does not stop the microprojectiles. They enter the target tissue. Getting nucleic acids into plant tissue by this means was first achieved using intact epidermal cells from onion as the target and RNA from tobacco mosaic virus or a DNA construct encoding chloramphenicol acetyltransferase. Expression of both these nucleic acids was detected. Biolistic transformation is now very widely used in plant and animal systems and has proved particularly useful in organelle transformation (see Section 9.7). The system can be used for situations requiring stable transformation or for transient expression work.

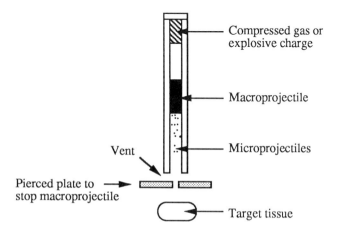

Figure 9.13 **The particle gun for biolistic transformation.**

9. 6. 5   Additional techniques

1. Viral transformation. Cloned DNA from the cauliflower mosaic virus (CaMV) causes viral infection when rubbed onto leaves of susceptible plants. Therefore, DNA can be inserted into the CaMV genome and then transferred into plants by rubbing onto the leaves. Although there appear to be significant restrictions on the sites where DNA can be inserted into the CaMV genome to retain viability, modifications to at least one of the genes, ORF II, are possible. In one example, a chimaeric molecule containing a sequence encoding a methotrexate-resistant version of the enzyme dihydrofolate reductase was introduced into turnip plants. The resulting plants produced the methotrexate-resistant enzyme and showed increased tolerance to methotrexate when it was sprayed onto their leaves. Although this demonstrated the feasibility of this approach under certain circumstances, the approach has not found general application – partly because of the narrow constraints on the sequences that the virus can accept without loss of viability, and partly because transformation is not always stable (presumably because the viral DNA is not integrated into the recipient).

2. Injection. Direct injection of DNA has also been used for insertion of DNA into plants. In one example, floral tillers of rye were microinjected with a construct containing a kanamycin resistance gene. After cross-pollination of 98 injected plants, 3,023 seeds were tested on medium that contained kanamycin and 7 apparently kanamycin-resistant seedlings were obtained. Two of the plants showed the aminoglycoside phosphotransferase activity encoded by the gene, and the probing of Southern blots with DNA from the plants indicated integration of the gene. Injection of DNA directly into individual cells has also been used, but these techniques are not yet widely used.

3. Other techniques. A wide range of other techniques have also been tried – including pollen transformation, injection into pollen tubes, and fusion with DNA-containing liposomes – with varying degrees of success. These approaches are not widely used, and in some cases there may be doubt about whether transformation has actually taken place.

9. 6. 6   Vectors

Incoming DNA is generally integrated into the host genome instead of existing as a stable extrachromosomal element. For *Agrobacterium*-mediated transformation, the vectors used contain the border repeats that are an important part of the transfer and integration processes as described in Section 9.6.1. In the other techniques, there need be no special sequences to direct integration. Homologous recombination is possible, if the incoming DNA contains sequences that are also represented in the genome; otherwise the DNA is integrated more or less at random. (It is quite probably not completely at random, but at present it is not possible to predict the sites.) This can pose problems of "position effects", in which the degree of expression of the foreign sequences varies widely between different transgenic plants as a consequence of where in the genome the DNA has been inserted.

The most widely used selectable marker for transformation is resistance to kanamycin or related antibiotics, such as neomycin and G418, conferred by the bacterial aminoglycoside phosphotransferase gene. This gene is generally used under the control of the promoter from the *nos* gene for nopaline synthase

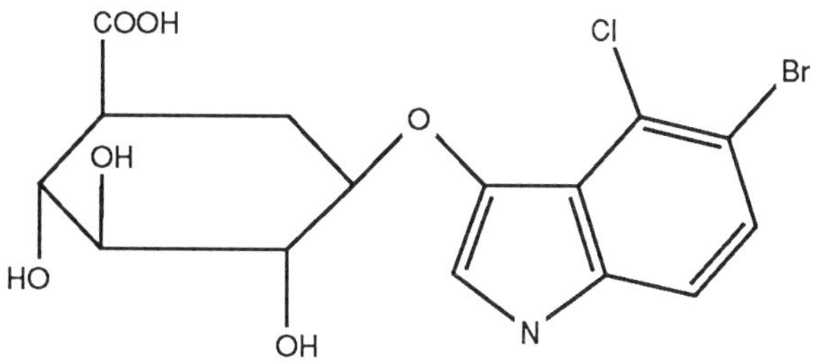

Figure 9.14 **Structure of X-Gluc (5-bromo-4-chloro-3-indolyl-ß-D glucuronide).**

(derived from a Ti plasmid). Although the *nos* gene is prokaryotic in origin, it is functional in plants, where it directs the synthesis of the opine, which is exploited by other *Agrobacterium* cells. Slight adjustments have been made to the sequence to improve expression, and this marker is contained within the "Bin" and related binary vectors. Less widely used selectable markers include genes conferring resistance to hygromycin, bialaphos (a herbicide), streptomycin, and methotrexate.

An important reporter gene is that for beta-glucuronidase. This enzyme will hydrolyse an artificial substrate, X-Gluc (5-bromo-4-chloro-3-indolyl-ß-D-glucuronide; Figure 9.14), to generate a blue pigment (analogous to the hydrolysis of X-Gal by beta-galactosidase). There is very little, if any, endogenous beta-glucuronidase activity in most plant tissues, but tissue sections can readily be stained for the enzyme with X-Gluc and plant extracts assayed for enzyme activity. The enzyme is particularly useful as a reporter gene product for assaying expression from modified control sequences that have been introduced into plant cells. Other substrates, such as 4-methyl-umbelliferyl-ß-D-glucuronide, can also be used. In this case, the product is measured fluorometrically. Other reporter genes include luciferase, which catalyses bioluminescent oxidation of luciferin and can be assayed by the light released; and chloramphenicol acetyltransferase. The latter can be assayed by its ability to transfer radioactive acetyl groups onto chloramphenicol.

One of the most widely used promoters is from the cauliflower mosaic virus (CaMV) and is called the 35S promoter, as it is responsible for the generation of a 35S transcript. It is constitutive and very active. Another important promoter is the *nos* promoter already mentioned. However, these promoters are relatively nonspecific, and for many applications it is desirable to restrict expression to certain tissues or certain conditions. A wide range of tissue-specific promoters are now being developed, such as the *rbcS* promoter, which is active in illuminated leaves and stems. Many constructs also incorporate terminators, to avoid readthrough from the inserted sequences into surrounding tissue. It may also prove important to take steps to avoid readthrough from surrounding tissue into the inserted sequences, which may be the cause of cosuppression, described in Section 7.7.2.

9. 6. 7 Applications

One of the favourite organisms for plant transformation work is *Nicotiana tabacum,* because the protocols for transformation and other manipulations are well established. However, the applications to other species, especially crop

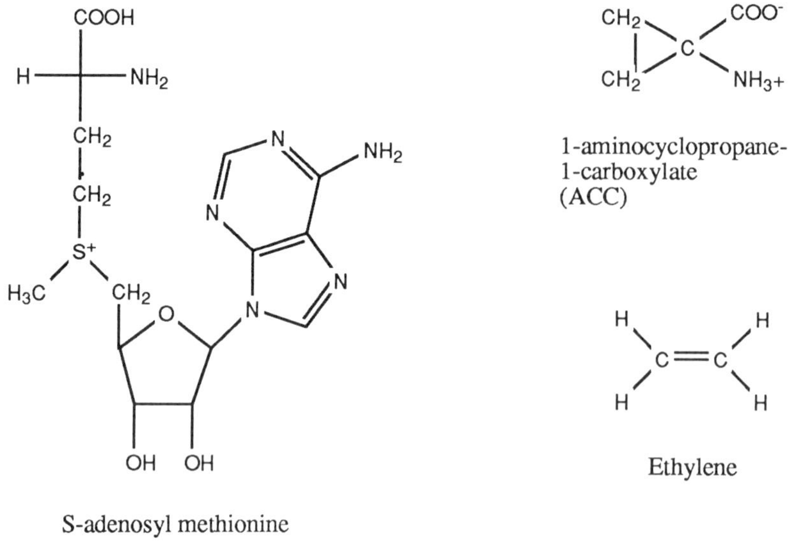

COOH

H————NH$_2$

CH$_2$

CH$_2$

S$^+$

H$_3$C   CH$_2$

O

OH   OH

S-adenosyl methionine

CH$_2$ COO$^-$

C

CH$_2$ NH$_3$+

1-aminocyclopropane-
1-carboxylate
(ACC)

NH$_2$

Ethylene

| S-adenosyl methionine $\longrightarrow$ ACC + 5' methylthio-adenosine | (ACC synthase) |
| ACC + 1/2 O$_2$ $\longrightarrow$ ethylene + HCN + CO$_2$+ H$_2$O | (ethylene-forming enzyme) |

Figure 9.15 **Synthesis of ethylene from S-adenosyl methionine via 1-aminocyclo-propane-1-carboxylate (ACC).**

plants, are very exciting. As well as the use in analysing gene expression and its control, there are many directly practical applications. For example:

1. **Herbicide resistance.** This can be achieved by causing plants to over-express the target protein for a herbicide in order to titrate the herbicide out, to produce a protein of modified sequence that is now resistant, or to produce an enzyme to detoxify the herbicide.

2. **Virus resistance.** This can be achieved by causing the plant to produce satellite RNA species that are found in attenuated strains of plant viruses (and that are responsible for the attenuation) or to overproduce viral coat-proteins, which inactivate incoming viral nucleic acids. Antisense and ribozyme techniques may also be useful.

3. **Insect resistance.** Many strains of the bacterium *Bacillus thuringiensis* produce proteinaceous insecticidal toxins during sporulation, and these can be used directly as insecticides. Genes for the toxins can be incorporated into plants, under appropriate promoters, to cause the plants to become insecticidal themselves.·

4. **Control of ripening.** Ripening in tomatoes depends on the production of and response to ethylene. This is produced from 1-aminocyclopropane-1-carboxylate (ACC) by the ethylene-forming enzyme. ACC is produced by ACC synthase

(Figure 9.15). Inactivation of expression of either of these enzymes by use of antisense RNA generates plants yielding fruit that do not ripen of their own accord (as they are unable to produce ethylene) but will do so if given exogenous ethylene.

5. Male sterility. Male-sterile plants (that do not produce viable pollen) are an important tool in plant breeding, to avoid self-pollination. Incorporation of a bacterial ribonuclease gene attached to a promoter specific for the tapetum (tissue surrounding the pollen sac, which is important in pollen development) leads to failure of pollen formation and results in male sterility.

6. Sensitivity to chilling. The sensitivity of plants to chilling depends to some extent on the degree of unsaturation of the fatty acids in the chloroplast membrane, and this in turn is influenced by the enzyme glycerol-3-phosphate acyltransferase in the chloroplast. Overexpression of this enzyme (with a suitable chloroplast-targeting peptide) can lead to plants with an increased resistance to damage by chilling.

9. 7 ORGANELLE TRANSFORMATION

The examples we have covered so far deal with the modification of the nuclear genome. However, eukaryotes contain one or two additional genomes, located in the mitochondrion and the chloroplast. These genomes encode a small but significant part of the polypeptides of those organelles. The mitochondrial genome encodes mainly polypeptides involved in oxidative phosphorylation, and the chloroplast genome encodes mainly polypeptides involved in the light reactions of photosynthesis, protein synthesis, and a limited number of other functions. In addition, both organelle genomes encode rRNAs and tRNAs. Mutations in mtDNA frequently result in the cells' inability to carry out oxidative phosphorylation, and we will see later that this has been exploited in mitochondrial transformation work.

Early attempts to manipulate organelle genomes included the use of *Agrobacterium* and direct DNA uptake, but they met with limited success. It was difficult to demonstrate DNA uptake conclusively and reproducibly. For some purposes, a different approach could be taken by fusing to a gene a sequence that encoded an organelle-targeting peptide and then inserting the modified gene into the nucleus, rather than into the organelle. An example of this was the engineering of tolerance in tobacco to the herbicide atrazine. This herbicide acts on one of the polypeptides of the reaction centre of Photosystem II, which is the product of the chloroplast *psbA* gene. A construct was made containing a mutant *psbA* gene (whose product was resistant to atrazine) from *Amaranthus* fused to a sequence encoding the transit peptide of the small subunit of ribulose *bis*-phosphate carboxylase. (This polypeptide is encoded in the nucleus, synthesized in the cytoplasm, and subsequently imported into the chloroplast. The transit peptide is a region at the amino-terminus of the protein, which directs import into the chloroplast and is subsequently removed proteolytically.) This hybrid gene, with a plant nuclear promoter attached, was introduced into the nucleus by *Agrobacterium*-mediated transformation. The PsbA protein was produced and imported into the chloroplast under the direction of the transit peptide, and the plants showed a significant level of atrazine resistance. Similar approaches can be used to target other polypeptides to the chloro-plast or to the mitochondrion as appropriate, and if the presence of the normal gene in the organelle is not a problem, inserting modified organelle genes into the nucleus may well be suitable. For direct modification of the chloroplast and mitochondrial genomes, the particle gun is used (see Section 9.6.4).

9. 7. 1 Chloroplasts

The first chloroplast manipulation experiments used a *Chlamydomonas* strain mutant in the chloroplast gene *atpB,* encoding the beta subunit of the ATP syn-thase, an important multisubunit complex required for the generation of ATP using light energy. The mutant had a partial deletion of this gene, rendering it unable to grow photosynthetically and therefore dependent on a suitable fixed carbon source, such as acetate, in its growth medium. Cells were bombarded with a plasmid containing the cloned wild-type gene, incubated for a while, then transferred to medium lacking a fixed carbon source and illuminated, thereby being selected for the restoration of photosynthetic competence. Photosynthetic colonies were obtained, containing an apparently normal beta subunit in the ATP synthase, and with the mutant region of chloroplast DNA replaced with the wild-type region, as demonstrated by Southern analysis. This replacement was pre-sumably the result of homologous recombination, and all copies of the chloroplast genome contained the wild-type sequence, since restriction fragments corresponding to the mutant could not be detected. The lack of any copies of the mutant allele is remarkable because the chloroplast DNA is present at a high copy number, and it indicates that the wild-type phenotype will be stable in the absence of continued selection. Other selections that have been successfully used in chloroplast transformation in *Chlamydomonas* include

  a. restoration of photosynthetic competence in strains mutant in *psbA* (for a component of Photosystem II) or *rbcL* (for the large subunit of the CO_2-fixing enzyme ribulose *bis*-phosphate carboxylase),

  b. resistance to streptomycin, spectinomycin, or erythromycin conferred by mutations in the 16S or 23S rRNA genes, and

  c. resistance to streptomycin or spectinomycin following acquisition of the bacterial *aadA* gene attached to chloroplast expression sequences.

The *aadA* gene for aminoglycoside adenyltransferase from the bacterium *Shigella flexneri* has also been used as a selectable marker for gene disruption. An advantage with the use of *Chlamydomonas* for transformation (and espe-cially for gene disruption) is that, unlike higher plants, the organism has a single chloroplast, and there is therefore no risk of getting cells containing a mixture of chloroplasts, some of which have been genetically altered and some of which have not. Such cells are said to be *heteroplasmic,* rather than *homoplasmic.* There is still the possibility of getting mixed populations of genomes within the single chloroplast, and this may occur if disruption of all copies of the gene would result in cell death. Chloroplast transformation by rapid mixing of proto-plasts with DNA and glass beads has also been reported.

Chloroplast transformation in higher plants is possible with antibiotic resis-tance conferred by 16S rRNA mutations or the *aadA* construct as selectable markers. As with *Chlamydomonas*, sequences are integrated at high efficiency by homologous recombination, although plasmids that incorporate a chloroplast origin of replication and are stably maintained extrachromosomally have been constructed. Transient expression of sequences forced into the chloroplast by the particle gun has also been exploited.

9. 7. 2 Mitochondria

For mitochondrial transformation, a slightly different approach from that used with chloroplasts was taken (Figure 9.16). It used *Saccharomyces cerevisiae* cells that were mutant in the nuclear *URA3* gene and in the mitochondrial *coxI* gene, encoding subunit I of cytochrome oxidase. The mitochondrial mutation renders the cells unable to carry out oxidative phosphorylation and, consequently, unable to grow on glycerol as a carbon source (as cells cannot grow on glycerol by fermentation alone). The cells were bombarded with particles carrying a mixture of DNAs containing wild-type *COXI* and *URA3* and selected for the acquisition of wild-type *URA3* but not, initially, wild-type *COXI*. Colonies that grew in the absence of exogenous uracil were then plated onto medium containing glycerol as the sole carbon source, to select for wild-type *COXI* cells – which were indeed obtained. It was argued that the initial selection for *URA3* acquisition would isolate those cells that had received DNA, and from these, the cells that had incorporated the mitochondrial DNA could be selected more easily. As with chloroplast transformation, it seemed that the wild-type sequences were integrated by homologous recombination to replace the defective sequences.

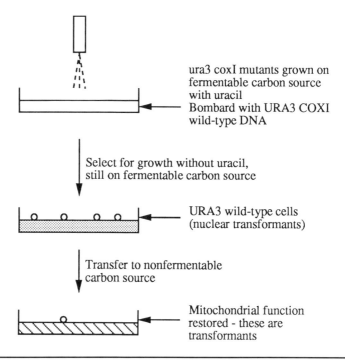

Figure 9.16 **Transformation of yeast mitochondria.** Selection takes place in two stages. In the first, nuclear transformants are selected. Transformants are then screened for mitochondrial transformation.

sion of the inserted sequence. Other approaches have also been taken; for example, using a nuclear polyhedrosis virus from *Bombyx mori*, then infecting silkworm larvae with the recombinant viruses and recovering protein from the haemolymph. Expression of proteins using nuclear polyhedrosis viruses is advantageous not only because it gives high protein yields, but also because a range of posttranslational modifications may be carried out that are carried out much less reliably (if at all) with prokaryotic and yeast systems. These modifications include glycosylation (O- and N-linked), phosphorylation, proteolytic processing, secretion, and acylation. One or more of these modifications may be required for the expressed protein to have biological activity.

However, the size of the viral genome presents a problem, as it is too large to be easily manipulated *in vitro*. A convenient solution is to use a system akin to the cointegrative vector system used with *Agrobacterium tumefaciens*. The baculovirus system requires a small plasmid termed the *transfer vector*. Figure 9.18 illustrates an example of a typical transfer vector that contains the following: sequences to allow propagation in *E. coli*; the polyhedrin gene promoter; the polyhedrin mRNA polyadenylation signal; and sequences that, in the virus, flanked both ends of the polyhedrin gene. The gene to be expressed is inserted adjacent to the polyhedrin promoter (which can be done to generate fusion proteins or intact proteins, depending on the vector used). The construct is then transfected into cultured insect cells, along with complete intact viral genomic

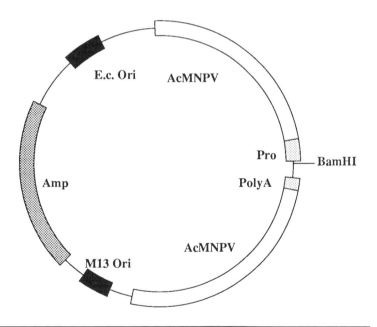

Figure 9.18 Plasmid pBacPAK1 (5.5 kb) from a baculovirus transfer vector system. Sequences can be inserted into the *Bam*HI site between the polyhedrin promoter (Pro) and the polyadenylation site (PolyA). Viral sequences on each side (AcMNPV) allow integration into a complete viral genome by recombination. The plasmid can be grown in *E. coli* using the origin (E.c. Ori) and ampicillin resistance marker (Amp), and there is an origin for single-stranded DNA synthesis (M13 Ori).

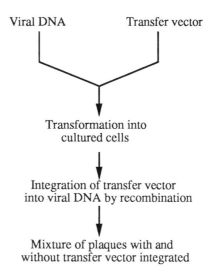

Figure 9.19 **Use of baculovirus viral and transfer vectors.**

DNA, giving rise to infection plaques in the host cells. The transfection can easily be accomplished by coprecipitation of the DNA onto the cells with calcium phosphate, or by incorporation of the DNA into liposomes that fuse with the insect cells. Once the DNA is inside the insect cells, homologous recombination can then take place, in which the polyhedrin gene from the intact viral genome is replaced with the region containing the foreign DNA. This recombination occurs between the sequences flanking the polyhedrin gene in the intact viral DNA and the corresponding homologous sequences in the transfer vector. Recombination generates a modified virus containing the foreign DNA. Plaques produced by the modified virus can be distinguished visually from plaques formed by the wild-type virus. Large quantities of cells can then be grown and infected with the modified virus (techniques for this are quite well developed). Within these infected cells, the polyhedrin promoter directs high levels of transcription of the inserted sequence. The presence of the polyadenylation signal ensures that the mRNA produced is polyadenylated. Large amounts of protein are synthesized, which can be harvested. The whole procedure is summarized in Figure 9.19.

Modifications. One potential difficulty with the baculovirus transfer vector system is the reliance on recombination. Various modifications have been made to alleviate this. Some transfer vectors contain a *lacZ* gene adjacent to the site for insertion of the sequences for expression. The expression in plaques of *lacZ* (detected using X-Gal) therefore indicates that the plaques contain recombinant viruses (i.e., ones including the transfer vector). This helps in detection of recombinants, but it does not increase their frequency. Note that this differs from the uses we have seen of *lacZ* so far, in which the cloning sites were located within the gene. Modifications to improve the recombination frequency include simply linearizing the DNA, on the grounds that this appears to make it more recom-

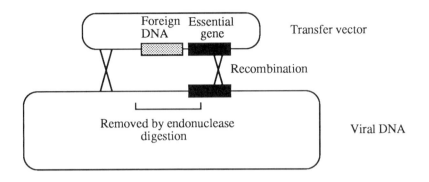

Figure 9.20 **Selection for recombination between virus and transfer vector when using a baculovirus system.** An essential region of the viral genome is removed by restriction endonuclease digestion. Intact functional virus can be regenerated by recombination with the transfer vector.

binogenic; and selection schemes whereby regions essential for viral growth are removed from the viral genome by restriction digestion and can only be reconstituted by recombination with the transfer vector (Figure 9.20). Thus, the only plaques formed should contain recombinant viruses (as only recombinant viruses have the complete gene needed to infect cells). Other modifications to the basic system include improvements to the cloning sites, incorporation of single-strand origins of replication, and so on, as we have seen with other systems.

9. 8. 2 *Drosophila*

Direct transformation of cultured *Drosophila* cells is possible, but for many applications we need to introduce genes into whole organisms. A convenient method for doing this is the microinjection of DNA into *Drosophila* embryos. They are injected at the pre-blastoderm stage, when the embryo contains a layer of nuclei that have not been separated into individual cells. This is called a *syncytium,* and injecting embryos at this stage means that many nuclei will be accessible to the incoming DNA. For reasons that will become clear, though, it is only the nuclei that will give rise to germ line cells (located at one end of the embryo) that acquire DNA stably. Embryos are then grown to maturity. The mature flies will be mosaic, with some of the germ line cells transgenic. Mating these flies produces progeny that are transgenic, but no longer mosaic.

In contrast to what happens in many other organisms, injected DNA will not integrate efficiently into the chromosomes of *Drosophila* unaided. It is therefore necessary to rely on a "natural" integration system that depends on transposable elements found in *Drosophila* called P elements. These are the basis of a phenomenon called *hybrid dysgenesis.* Under the action of a transposase that is also encoded by the P element, they will insert themselves at random into the DNA of *Drosophila* germ line cells. An artificial P element that does not encode transposase, but does have its site of action, can also become integrated if the transposase is provided by a helper P element that is also present. (This is reminiscent of the binary vector systems used with *Agrobacterium.*) So in genetic manipulation of *Drosophila* (Figure 9.21), the sequences to be inserted are first incorporated into a modified P element, which needs to contain only a genetic

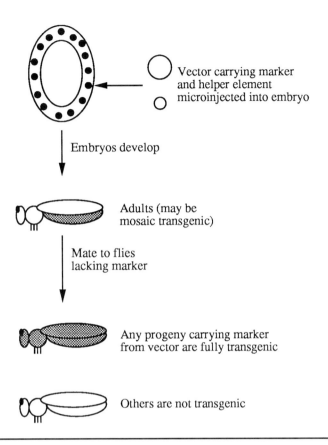

Figure 9.21 Genetic manipulation of Drosophila. Mosaic transgenic flies are generated by insertion of an artificial P element into germ line cells. Progeny derived from transgenic germ cells are fully transgenic.

marker and those *cis*-acting sequences needed for transposase activity. This element is then microinjected into pre-blastoderm embryos, together with a helper P element DNA. Microinjection is carried out using a micromanipulator and tiny glass pipettes, although particle bombardment can also be used. Within the syncytial embryo, some of the P element DNAs will find themselves in the region that will ultimately develop into the germ line. During that development, the helper element directs the production of the transposase protein, and this protein causes the integration of the modified P element into the germ line genome. Transgenic gametes will be produced when the fly is mature. But note that not all the germ line cells will necessarily be transgenic, and the rest of the fly will not be – it is a mosaic. To generate a fully transgenic fly, we have to mate the mosaic and obtain progeny flies. Progeny flies that are produced from a nontransgenic gamete from the mosaic will not be transgenic. Progeny formed from a transgenic gamete will be fully transgenic and not mosaic. These flies are identifiable by the presence of the genetic marker on the P element. The site of integration of the P element seems to be more or less random, as with *Agrobacterium* T-DNA insertion. Insertion is due to a specific recombinase activity, rather than general homologous recombination.

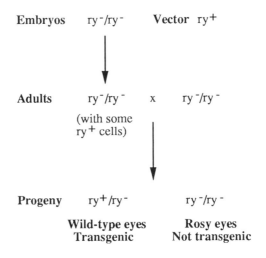

Figure 9.22 **Use of the rosy gene in manipulation of *Drosophila*.**

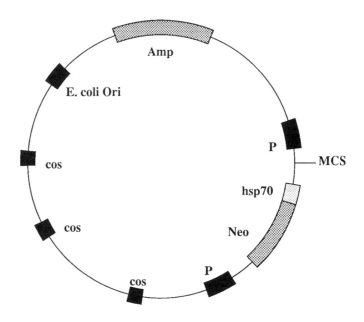

Figure 9.23 ***Drosophila* vector cosPneo (9.2 kb).** The boxes (P) indicate the P element ends, and therefore the region transferred. There are a selectable marker for use in *Drosophila* (a neomycin resistance gene [Neo] under the control of the *Drosophila hsp70* promoter); and *cos* sites, a selectable marker (Amp), and an origin of replication for use in *E. coli* before transfer into the *Drosophila* host.

1. **Markers.** The first marker used for transformation with P elements was the wild type *rosy* gene, *ry*. This encodes xanthine dehydrogenase, which carries out a step in the synthesis of eye pigments. Wild-type flies have brick-red eyes, whereas *rosy* mutants have dark crimson to brown eyes. So if the host fly embryo that is injected and the fly that it is subsequently mated with are both *ry⁻*, and if the vector carries the wild-type gene, transgenic progeny flies can be identified as those with the wild-type eye colour, as shown in Figure 9.22. A disadvantage of *rosy* is that the gene is rather large. A smaller marker is the alcohol dehydrogenase *adh* gene. Wild-type flies can be selected by their resistance to ethanol supplied in the food; ethanol is toxic to *adh⁻* mutants. Other markers used include the bacterial neomycin phosphotransferase gene attached to a *Drosophila* heat shock promoter, selectable by inclusion of the antibiotic G418 or neomycin in the food; the eye marker *white* (affecting colour); and another eye marker, *rough* (affecting morphology).

2. **Vectors.** As well as a marker, a vector should contain the appropriate *cis*-acting sites for the transposition process. A vector may also need a promoter to direct expression of inserted sequences. The promoter from the heat shock gene *hsp70* is often used for this. There are also more complex vectors, such as that shown in Figure 9.23, which can function as a cosmid in *E. coli*.

3. **Helpers and hosts.** Various helper elements are available. The helper elements must encode a functional transposase, and some have been modified to try to increase transposase production. Many helper elements have mutations in their own *cis*-acting transposition sequences, so that although they can direct the transposition of other sequences, they cannot be incorporated into the transgenic flies themselves. If they were incorporated, it would lead to genetic instability as the elements transposed in subsequent generations. The host strain should not contain any integrated P elements, because these might also cause instability. The host must carry suitable mutations for the subsequent detection of incorporated DNA.

9.9 MAMMALS

The other animal group we will look at in detail is mammals, although many of the techniques outlined here can be applied to other vertebrates, such as amphibians and fish. There are three kinds of genetic manipulation that we might need to carry out; they involve cultured cells, restricted areas of intact organisms, or whole individuals.

9.9.1 Cultured cells

1. **Selectable markers.** The first transformations in mammalian systems were achieved with cultured cells from humans suffering from the Lesch-Nyhan syndrome, which is caused by a deficiency of the enzyme hypoxanthine-guanine phosphoribosyl transferase, or HGPRT. Cells deficient in HGPRT die in a selective medium containing hypoxanthine, aminopterin, and thymidine (called HAT medium; Figure 9.24). This is because aminopterin blocks the pathway for endogenous synthesis of the purines needed for production of nucleic acids. An alternative pathway allows synthesis of purines from hypoxanthine, but this requires the enzyme HGPRT and so cannot operate in HGPRT⁻ cells. So HGPRT⁻ cells are unable to make nucleic acids in HAT medium and will die;

PURINES

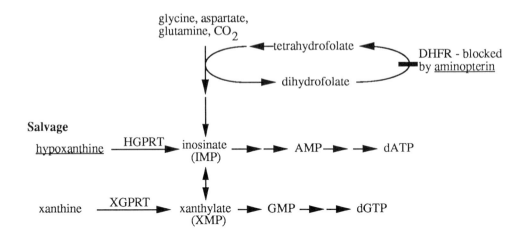

PYRIMIDINES

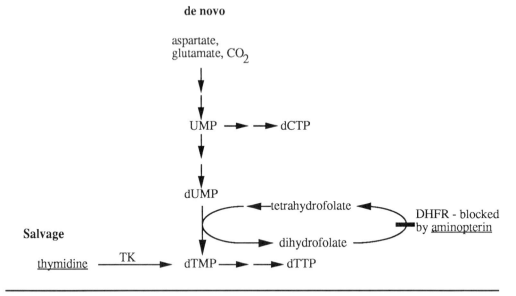

Figure 9.24 **HAT selection.** Compounds present in HAT medium are underlined. Aminopterin blocks the *de novo* synthesis of purine and pyrimidine nucleotides; synthesis from hypoxanthine and synthesis from thymidine require functional HGPRT and TK enzymes respectively.

wild-type cells are able to make nucleic acids and will live. Precipitation of wild-type DNA onto the HGPRT⁻ cells in the presence of calcium phosphate led to DNA uptake and stable transformation. Similar results could be obtained with cells deficient in thymidine kinase (TK). They are also killed in HAT medium. Pyrimidine synthesis is also blocked by aminopterin, and utilization of the thymidine supplied in the HAT medium (Figure 9.24) requires a functional thymidine kinase. Transformation of TK⁻ cells with DNA containing a functional TK gene gave rise to cells that were able to survive in HAT medium.

So suitable treatment of cultured cells can lead to uptake and expression of exogenous DNA. In addition to HGPRT and TK genes, commonly used selectable markers for mammalian cell transformation include:

a. resistance to aminoglycoside antibiotics, conferred by the bacterial neomycin phosphotransferase gene attached to a suitable promoter

b. resistance to methotrexate, conferred by a gene that produces a resistant version of the enzyme dihydrofolate reductase, which is the normal site of action of methotrexate

c. overexpressing glutamine synthetase genes, which allow cells to continue to make glutamine from exogenous glutamate and ammonia in the presence of the glutamine synthetase inhibitor methionine sulphoximine

d. the bacterial xanthine-guanine phosphoribosyl transferase (XGPRT) gene, which allows HGPRT⁻ cells to utilize xanthine for purine nucleotide biosynthesis

e. resistance to toxic adenosine nucleosides, such as 9-ß-D-xylofuranosyl adenine conferred by adenosine deaminase

f. resistance to difluoromethylornithine, conferred by ornithine decarboxylase

With the last three markers, it is necessary to use cells that are deficient in the corresponding enzyme to allow selection for the marker. Selection for a particular marker gene can sometimes result in amplification of the number of copies of the gene in the target cells, which may be useful, although the amplification is not always stable in the absence of continued selection. The *absence* of a functional thymidine kinase gene can be selected by the use of gancyclovir or 5-bromodeoxyuridine, which kill cells after metabolism by TK.

As in some other systems, cotransformation is often observed, where cells that have been selected for acquisition of one marker are frequently found to have acquired an unlinked and unselected marker that was supplied at the same time. This means that a selected marker does not necessarily have to be on the same piece of DNA as other transforming sequences.

2. Transformation methods and hosts. Calcium phosphate coprecipitation (the first transformation method used successfully with mammalian cells) is easily achieved by mixing a solution containing the DNA with solutions containing phosphate ions and calcium ions. This results in the formation of a very fine precipitate of calcium phosphate, particles of which are probably taken up by the cells phagocytotically, with the DNA included passively in the process.

Further treatment with glycerol or dimethyl sulphoxide may improve the efficiency of uptake. DNA can conveniently be introduced into cells by many other techniques, including treatment with DEAE-dextran; fusion with liposomes, *E. coli* protoplasts, or red blood cell *ghosts* (cells whose contents have been removed and replaced, by swelling and shrinking in solutions of suitable osmotic strengths) containing the DNA; electroporation; microprojectile bombardment; and laser permeabilization. Many cultured cell lines can be used, including COS cells (derived from kidney cells from African green monkeys and transformed with a defective SV40), Chinese hamster ovary (CHO) cells, HeLa cells, mouse 3T3 cells, and many others.

3. Vectors. There are many vectors available. Some will replicate effectively in cultured cells, allowing extrachromosomal retention. Others will not, and they must therefore be used in transient expression systems unless they can integrate into the chromosome. There is a range of expression vectors, although they will, of course, be unnecessary if one wishes simply to test the activity of particular promoter constructs in transformed cells. Overexpression of the cloned sequences, on the other hand, can be used for many purposes, including tests of biological function and library screening. Selection for complementation in cells from lines deficient in a particular function allows the identification of cells containing the equivalent cloned gene or cDNA. This has been used, for example, to recover cDNAs for genes involved in DNA repair, by complementation of repair-deficient cell lines. If an overexpressed protein is expressed at the cell surface, it may be possible to select appropriate cells using some kind of *panning* affinity technique using antibodies or a ligand (see "Ligand binding by the expressed protein" in Section 5.2.2). Use of mammalian cells for panning (when trying to isolate genes for particular mammalian proteins) has the advantage over systems such as phage display that the protein is more likely to achieve its correct conformation in the membrane and undergo any necessary posttranslational modification. Clearly, the details of the selection methods used will depend on the particular function of the protein in question and the nature of the cells expressing it.

Many vectors are based on the virus SV40. This can replicate successfully in certain cell types, such as those derived from the African green monkey, which are said to be *permissive*. Additional virus particles can be produced, which will go on and infect other cells, although eventually lysis will take place. In *nonpermissive* cells, virus replication does not take place, although the viral DNA can still be expressed. If selection for the incoming sequences is imposed, then the only way they can be maintained in nonpermissive cells is by integration.

SV40 normally produces two sets of transcripts, denoted *early* and *late*. They are initiated divergently from near the origin of replication, and production of the early transcripts is stimulated by two 72-base-pair enhancer sequences. Both sets of transcripts are spliced and polyadenylated. It seems that splicing of transcripts is necessary for efficient expression. Transcripts that have not been through a splicing process are not expressed efficiently, even if introns have been artificially removed from the DNA. So if vectors are to be based upon insertion of sequences into the regions covered by the early or late transcripts, it is important not to disrupt the splicing sites even if the inserted sequences themselves do not contain introns. An example of such a vector is

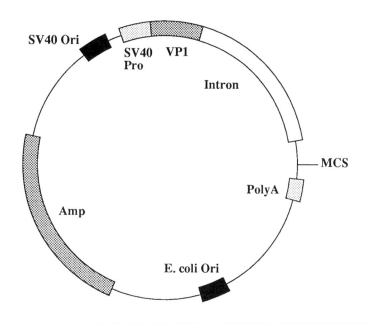

Figure 9.25 Plasmid pSVL (4.9 kb). The vector contains the SV40 late promoter (SV40 Pro) and part of the region encoding a viral polypeptide (VP1), with an intron and polyadenylation site (PolyA) associated with VP1. There are SV40 and prokaryotic origins, and a prokaryotic selectable marker (Amp).

pSVL, shown in Figure 9.25. This shuttle vector contains pBR322 sequences (from which a "poison" sequence causing reduced replication efficiency has been deleted) that include the ampicillin resistance gene and the origin of replication. SV40 sequences include the origin of replication; the late promoter; a region, transcribed from that promoter, that includes intron material; and the polyadenylation site. DNA is inserted after the intron, allowing efficient splicing and polyadenylation. Replication would be possible in permissive cells, giving a high copy number, were it not for the fact that the vector lacks the coding sequence for the T protein (a product of early viral transcription), which is also required for replication. So in the absence of T, maintenance of the plasmid is possible only by integration. Replication in permissive cells and maintenance extrachromosomally are possible if the cells are co-infected with a helper virus, or if the cells produce the T protein themselves. This is the case with COS cells (described earlier). These cells will support a high copy number (and, in principle, high expression levels) of SV40-based vectors, although in some cases the high copy number is not retained indefinitely. Control of copy number is possible using a variant of COS cells that produces a temperature-sensitive T protein. Complementation to produce more virus particles (rather than just replication of viral DNA) would require, in addition, the provision of the late viral VP1, VP2, and VP3 proteins, which can be provided by a helper virus. Packaging places constraints on the size of insert DNA that can be accommodated.

Another widely used virus is the vaccinia virus, a member of the pox virus family. It has a large genome, nearly 200 kb, but can accept at least 25 kb of extra foreign DNA. The virus encodes its own RNA polymerase, which is functional in the cytoplasm of infected cells, where the virus replicates. Because of the size of the viral genome, recombinants are generated *in vivo* in infected cells by recombination between a suitable plasmid, into which the sequences of interest have been inserted, and a parental virus strain (as with the baculoviruses). Plasmid is transfected into cells carrying the virus, and recombination integrates the plasmid into the virus. Techniques are available for the selection of recombinant viruses, for example, by conferring the ability to replicate in suitable cell lines. Recombinant vaccinia viruses can be used as live vaccines, as well as for the expression of genes in cultured cell lines.

Figure 9.26 gives an example of a plasmid vector, pAbT4586, for use in the vaccinia system. This contains two viral promoters (P7.5K and P40K) with cloning sites adjacent to them, a modified *lacZ* marker gene, and nonfunctional viral thymidine kinase sequences. The plasmid integrates into the viral genome by recombination across the thymidine kinase sequences, rendering the virus TK⁻ because the endogenous viral TK gene is thereby disrupted. TK⁻ host cells are used, which can grow in the presence of 5-bromodeoxyuridine (see "Selectable markers"). Host cells carrying nonrecombinant virus will be TK⁺ and will be killed by 5-bromodeoxyuridine. Cells carrying a recombinant virus will still be TK⁻ and will survive in the presence of 5-bromodeoxyuridine. Virus plaques will be blue in the presence of X-Gal because of the beta-galactosidase gene.

Retroviruses are also very useful for genetic manipulation. They have the advantages that they will infect susceptible cells with very high efficiency and bring about stable integration into the target cell genome. An example, LNSX,

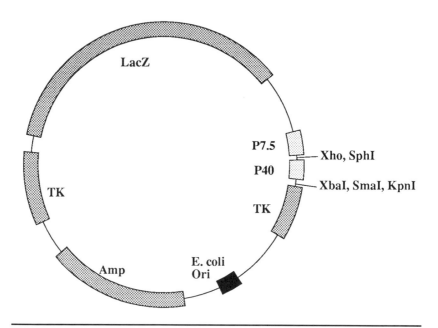

Figure 9.26 **Plasmid pAbT4586 (7.8 kb), containing two vaccinia virus promoters (P7.5 and P40).** The viral thymidine kinase (TK) sequences allow integration into a viral genome by recombination.

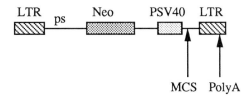

Figure 9.27 **Part of the retrovirus-based vector LNSX.** (For simplicity, only the retroviral part of the vector is shown.) LTR=long terminal repeat; ps=packaging signal.

is shown in Figure 9.27. This retrovirus contains a neomycin resistance gene as a selectable marker and contains a promoter (in this case, the SV40 early promoter) adjacent to a multiple cloning site. It is usually combined with a prokaryotic plasmid to function as a shuttle vector. It does not encode viral proteins, so it cannot itself integrate directly into a host genome. After any construction work in a prokaryotic host has been completed, the retroviral vector is transfected as naked DNA into mammalian cells infected with a helper retrovirus. In these cells, RNA transcripts are produced from the incoming retroviral vector DNA, and these are then packaged into retroviral particles containing the proteins (encoded by the helper retrovirus), such as reverse transcriptase, needed for subsequent infection of target cells. The resulting packaged viruses can then be used to infect other target cells efficiently, resulting in reverse transcription of the retroviral DNA and stable integration of DNA into the recipient cell genome. It is important to stop the helper retrovirus from being packaged as well. This can be done by three methods (Figure 9.28): deletion of the packaging signal in the helper genome; deletion of multiple parts of the helper genome; or division of the helper genome into several different pieces.

Other viruses used as a basis for vector construction include polyoma virus, which is closely related to SV40, both being members of the papovavirus family; Epstein-Barr virus; and bovine papilloma virus (Figure 9.29). There is considerable interest in the development of mammalian artificial chromosomes (MACs, analogous to YACs), although these are at an early stage at present.

4. Constitutive promoters. Promoters used in any of the vectors described can be divided conveniently into a number of groups: those that are constitutive, and those that are induced in response to various signals. Constitutive promoters are frequently derived from viruses. They include the SV40 promoters, the Rous sarcoma virus promoter, the adenovirus major late promoter, and the cytomegalovirus immediate early promoter. Hybrid promoters exist, containing elements from – for example – cytomegalovirus and human immunodeficiency virus. Enhancers are often included, too, and frequently-used ones are derived from SV40, Rous sarcoma virus, and cytomegalovirus. However, some enhancers confer a significant degree of tissue specificity and may be unsuitable as general constitutive expression vectors.

5. Glucocorticoid-inducible promoters. A widely used glucocorticoid-responsive promoter comes from the long terminal repeat (LTR) of the mouse

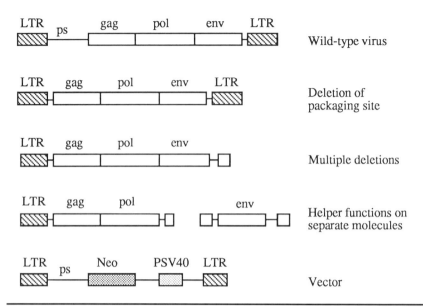

Figure 9.28 **Strategies for avoiding packaging of helper retrovirus.** The top and bottom diagrams show wild-type virus and a typical vector molecule (see Figure 9.27) respectively. The middle diagrams show three helper retrovirus systems that can provide all the functions for vector packaging, but cannot themselves be packaged. (Only the retroviral part of vectors are shown.) gag, pol, and env are retroviral genes. ps is the packaging signal.

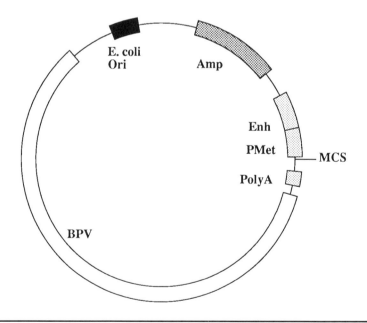

Figure 9.29 **Plasmid pBPV (12.5 kb), based on bovine papilloma virus (BPV).** There is an enhancer (Enh) derived from the Moloney murine sarcoma virus, a metallothionein promoter (PMet), and an SV40 splicing and polyadenylation site (PolyA).

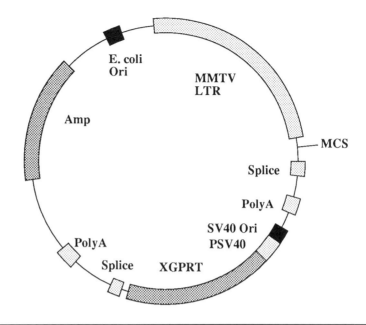

Figure 9.30 **Plasmid pMSG (7.6 kb).** This contains a mouse mammary tumour virus LTR sequence (MMTV LTR), containing a glucocorticoid-inducible promoter. There are also SV40 splice and polyadenylation sites (Splice, PolyA). An SV40 origin-promoter region (SV40 Ori and PSV40) drives expression of a bacterial XGPRT gene for use as a selectable marker in mammalian cells. There are also splice and polyadenylation sites to aid the XGPRT expression, and a prokaryotic origin and marker for propagation in *E. coli*.

mammary tumour virus (MMTV). The LTR contains a glucocorticoid-responsive element to which a hormone-receptor complex can bind, activating transcription from the promoter. An example of a vector based on this is pMSG (Figure 9.30), which includes elements from SV40 and pBR322, and a selectable marker (the *E. coli* xanthine-guanine phosphoribosyl transferase gene under the control of the SV40 early promoter). Induction of expression requires treatment with a suitable hormone (or analogue), such as dexamethasone, and the presence of the hormone receptor in the cells. This can be provided either by using a cell type that is already hormone responsive, or by artificial expression in the cells of a receptor protein gene. This approach can be modified to improve expression further by incorporation of several copies of the glucocorticoid response element in the vector.

6. Metal-inducible promoters. Another important group of promoters comes from the genes for metallothioneins (Figure 9.29). These are a group of proteins rich in cysteine residues, which chelate heavy metals to reduce their toxicity. The promoters can be induced by treatment of cells with heavy metal ions, such as zinc and cadmium. Inducibility depends on the presence of a binding site for a control protein, and this binding site can be incorporated into other promoters, too. Use of metal-inducible promoters has two disadvantages: the heavy metal ions may be damaging to the cells involved; and the control is not particularly tight, so that there may be significant levels of expression in the absence of the metal ions.

7. **Heat shock–inducible promoters.** When cells are exposed to a heat shock, a specific set of genes is activated. This is mediated by the binding of a transcription factor to an element upstream from the promoters. This element can be used either with its normal promoter or in association with others to give controlled expression.

8. **Other considerations.** The amount of expression of DNA inserted into a vector will not depend only on the promoter used. If sequences are integrated into the host genome, their chromosomal location is important. Flanking the inserted gene by *A elements* (or Scaffold Attachment Regions), which are sites for attachment of the chromatin to the chromosomal scaffold, may help to reduce the position effects resulting from chromosomal location. The presence of introns in the sequences to be expressed is also important (see "Vectors" in this section), as are other factors, such as polyadenylation of the transcript and efficient translation initiation.

9. 9. 2   Restricted areas of intact organisms

Introduction of DNA into a small region of tissue from an intact organism may be useful, for example in studies involving expression, or in models for gene therapy. The principles for vector construction already outlined apply, although expression will usually be transient. DNA can be introduced into the tissue by microprojectile bombardment. Direct injection may be suitable for some tissues, such as muscle, which forms a syncytium. Introduction by inhalation of an aerosol of DNA-containing liposomes may allow treatment of cystic fibrosis, in which a mutation in the gene for a chloride transporter compromises lung function. Removal of cells from an organism, modification, and reintroduction may also be used to generate a mosaic transgenic organism.

9. 9. 3   Whole organisms

The selectable markers and promoters already discussed can also be used for generating whole organisms that are transgenic. There are three main methods, summarized in Figure 9.31. One is to isolate one-cell embryos (at which stage they are in the oviduct) and microinject DNA directly into the pronucleus. The embryos are then returned to a foster mother's oviduct, where development takes place. A second approach is to treat cleavage-stage embryos *in vitro* with recombinant retroviruses and then return them to the uterus of a foster mother. A third approach exploits the ability to grow and manipulate embryonic stem cells (ES cells) from the inner cell mass of a developing blastocyst. These pluripotent cells can be genetically modified *in vitro* and then reinjected into the blastocoel of a developing embryo. The injected embryo is then transferred to a foster mother's uterus. Although the ES cells will colonize the embryo, it will not be composed entirely of ES-derived cells, and the resulting animals will be chimaeric. Some ES-derived cells will become incorporated into the germ line. Matings with such animals can then generate progeny that are transgenic and not chimaeric, if a progeny animal is produced from a transgenic gamete. Producing transgenic individuals in this way is analogous to the generation of transgenic *Drosophila* described in Section 9.8.2. Use of suitable genetic markers, such as coat colour when mice are used, allows chimaeric individuals to be identified easily. Very large stretches of DNA can be acquired. Even YACs can be introduced – by microinjection or by fusion with yeast spheroplasts – and

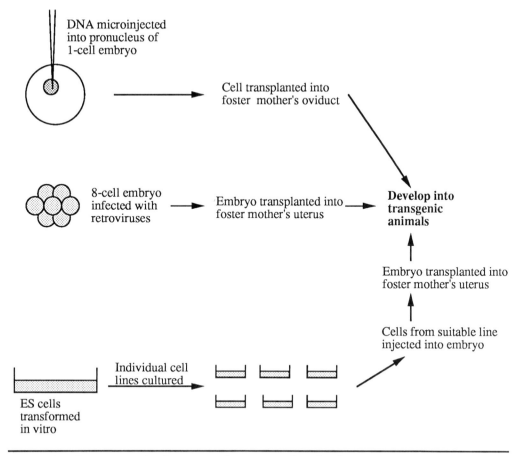

Figure 9.31 **Three strategies for generating transgenic animals.**

integrated with little or no rearrangement. Mammalian artificial chromosomes afford similar possibilities.

The use of the three approaches described for the random integration of incoming DNA is relatively straightforward. To bring about expression of incoming sequences, the usual considerations about promoters, polyadenylation, and so forth, must be applied. There are two developments of the standard techniques that we should look at in more detail: *trapping* and *gene targeting*. Trapping is a way of detecting when DNA has been inserted into a particular type of gene – perhaps a gene that is active at a certain developmental stage or in a particular tissue type. Gene targeting is the process of obtaining insertion of incoming DNA into homologous sites in the chromosome, rather than at random.

1. Trapping. The simplest trapping experiments use a vector containing a promoterless reporter gene, which functions only if it is integrated near a functional promoter. This is sometimes called *promoter trapping,* and it is analogous to the use of promoter probe vectors described in Section 5.3.1. There are other techniques, such as *enhancer trapping* (Figure 9.32a), which allows one to detect when a vector has integrated near an enhancer as the integration leads to enhanced expression of a gene on the vector. *Gene trapping* uses slightly more

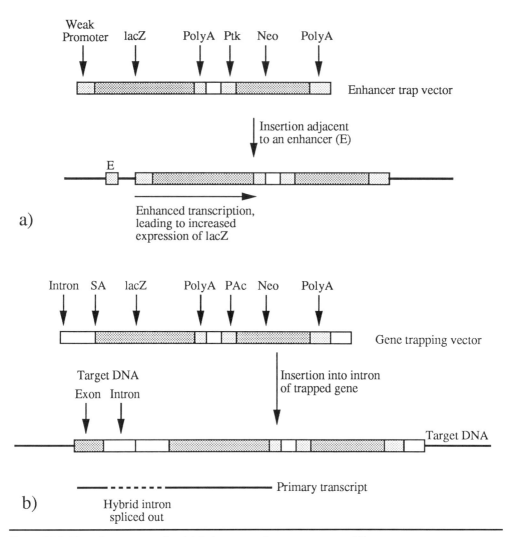

Figure 9.32 Trapping vectors. Panel **(a)** shows an enhancer trap vector. The neomycin resistance gene under the control of the thymidine kinase promoter (Ptk) allows selection for integration of the vector. In the cases where the vector has integrated near an enhancer (E), there will be enhanced expression of the *lacZ* gene on the vector. Panel **(b)** shows a gene trapping vector. The neomycin resistance gene under the control of the actin promoter (PAc) allows selection for integration of the vector. In the cases where the vector has integrated within an intron (as shown), a transcript will be produced that contains a hybrid intron (dotted line) – part coming from the target DNA sequence and part from the intron in the vector. The hybrid intron will be spliced out using the splice acceptor site in the vector (SA), giving a fusion between the target DNA exon and the *lacZ* of the vector.

complex vectors (Figure 9.32b) and allows one to detect insertion into an intron. In gene trapping, the reporter sequence (such as a promoterless part of *lacZ*) is preceded by part of an intron, with a splice acceptor site at the intron-*lacZ* junction. Having the splice acceptor site means that the *lacZ* sequence can be expressed when the vector is inserted into an intron (assuming the maintenance of the reading frame between the preceding exon and the inserted *lacZ* gene). Beta-galactosidase activity can easily be detected by staining the tissue with X-Gal. This staining allows easy detection of trapped genes that are active in particular tissues or developmental stages. Because the beta-galactosidase activity is not directly selectable, trapping vectors that use it as the reporter also need a selectable marker, such as neomycin phosphotransferase, to select initially just for integration events. Once a promoter, enhancer, or gene has been trapped in this way, the presence of the vector can be used as a tag to recover the trapped sequence from a library, as with transposon tagging (Section 5.2.3).

2. **Gene targeting.** If it is simply sufficient that a sequence be expressed in a transgenic organism, then it will not be necessary to ensure integration of the DNA at the normal chromosomal location. For some purposes, though, it may be neceessary to ensure such integration, perhaps to improve the regulation of expression of integrated DNA or to disrupt an endogenous gene. Obtaining integration at a particular site is called *gene targeting,* and it can be achieved using ES cells. Targeting relies on the fact that in ES cells, homologous recombination can take place between incoming DNA and the chromosome at the site of the corresponding sequences. The principle is that ES cells are screened after transformation for "correct" recombination, and only those that have undergone a suitable integration event are then injected into a developing embryo. Integration events may be insertional, involving a single crossover; or replacement, involving two crossovers, as described in Section 7.7.1. Selection for acquisition of the incoming DNA can be achieved quite easily – for example, by selection for a marker such as neomycin or G418 resistance. However, the difficulty is that – although homologous recombination can take place – nonhomologous recombination will also take place, causing sequences to be integrated at other sites. Further screening therefore has to be done after the initial neomycin selection for transformation, in order to identify those cells where homologous insertion has taken place.

In early experiments this screening was done by Southern blotting, using DNA from cultures derived from individual transformed cells. Screening many cell lines this way is laborious, and this approach has been superseded by PCR analysis. Homologous integration of sequences gives rise to fragments of predictable size when Southern blots are probed, or products of predictable size when PCR is used. The cells in which homologous recombination has taken place can then be used to generate transgenic organisms.

An example of gene targeting (Figure 9.33) is the disruption of the *Prn-p* gene, which encodes a protein found on the surface of neurons and certain other cell types, and which has been implicated in the disease scrapie. A linear fragment was constructed containing the neomycin phosphotransferase-coding region under the control of the thymidine kinase promoter from herpes simplex virus, flanked by *Prn-p* sequences. Cells were transformed with the fragment, and neomycin resistance selected. DNA from several different transformed cell lines was screened by PCR using one primer from within the neomycin phosphotransferase gene and one primer from a region of the *Prn-p* locus not present on the incoming DNA (see Figure 9.33). Only cells that had integrated the incoming DNA at the homologous position should give a PCR product – one, in this case, of 850 base pairs. This integration was then verified by Southern blotting, and cells were reintroduced into mouse blastocysts to produce chimaeric transgenic mice, which were then crossed with other mice to produce transgenic heterozygotes. Heterozygotes could then be crossed to produce homozygotes for the disrupted gene (which appeared surprisingly and disappointingly normal).

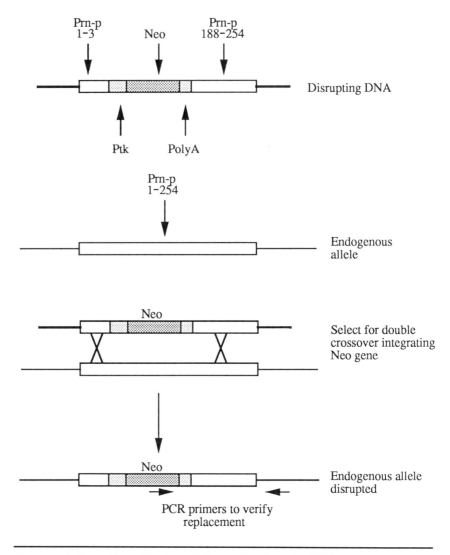

Figure 9.33 **Gene disruption in an ES cell.** The disrupting DNA contains a neomycin resistance gene (with a thymidine kinase promoter and a polyadenylation site) replacing codons 4–187 of the prion protein (Prn-p) gene. Integration of the Neo gene at the chromosomal site of the *Prn-p* gene can be demonstrated by the formation of a correctly sized PCR product using appropriate primers.

   The frequency of homologous recombination can be low compared to random integration, so it is useful to be able to select for the former. An example of selection for homologous recombination, involving two different rounds of selection, is summarized in Figure 9.34. The incoming DNA contains two markers. Selection of cells that have acquired the first (in this case, resistance to neomycin or G418) identifies those that have integrated DNA. The second marker is placed so that it is lost when integration is homologous, but is likely to be retained when it is not (because incorporation of molecules by nonhomologous recombination usually happens from the free ends). The second round of

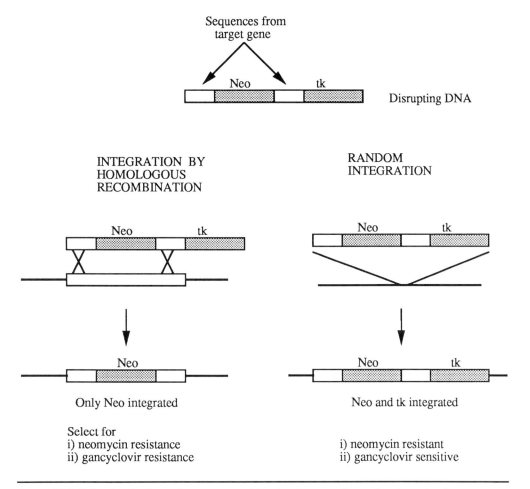

Figure 9.34 Selection for homologous recombination in gene disruption. Incoming disrupting DNA carries neomycin resistance and thymidine kinase markers. Homologous recombination between the chromosome and the sequences flanking the neomycin resistance gene does not integrate the thymidine kinase gene; random integration (stimulated by the free end of the molecule) does.

screening requires selection for cells that have *not* acquired the second marker, which in this case is the herpes simplex virus thymidine kinase gene. Expression of the gene renders cells sensitive to the nucleoside analogue gancyclovir (see Section 9.9.1), so cells that are resistant to both neomycin and gancyclovir are likely to have had a targeted disruption.

Sometimes it is desirable to make very minor changes to a target gene, without incorporating a selectable marker at that site, in case the marker disturbs expression. One approach relies on the fact that cells that have incorporated DNA at one site are likely to have also incorporated unlinked sequences at a different site (cotransformation). Cells are cotransformed with DNA bearing the mutated form of the target gene and with separate molecules bearing a selectable marker. Cells that have acquired the selectable marker by random integration are identified and then screened (e.g., by PCR) for co-acquisition of the mutation by homologous recombination at the target site.

3. Applications. The applications of transgenic animal technology are clearly extremely broad. For example, for studies on gene regulation, transgenic animals obviously provide a more realistic system than does the use of cultured cells. The genetic modification of farm animals may allow improved yield. A number of pharmaceutically important polypeptides have been produced in milk, by expressing them under the control of promoters active in the mammary gland. One of the most exciting prospects is the replacement of a wide range of defective genes in the relevant tissues in individuals suffering from defined genetic disorders.

References
and Further
Reading

This is not meant to be an exhaustive list of references in support of the material in the book. It is intended to be a collection of articles to offer further information on the topics discussed. Many of the companies marketing enzymes and other reagents for recombinant DNA work (such as Boehringer Mannheim, Clontech, Pharmacia, Promega, and Stratagene) provide very detailed and informative descriptions of vectors and techniques in their catalogues. Detailed references to these are not given here, but they may well be found very helpful.

Chapter 1

Kessler, C. & Manta, V. (1990). Specificity of restriction endonucleases and DNA modification methyltransferases. *Gene,* 92: 1–248.

Sambrook, J., Fritsch, E.F. & Maniatis, T. (1989). *Molecular cloning: A laboratory manual* (see especially Chapters 5 and 6). 2nd Edition, Cold Spring Harbor Laboratory Press.

Wilson, G.G. & Murray, N.E. (1991). Restriction and modification systems. *Annual Reviews of Genetics,* 25: 585–627.

Chapter 2

Hanahan, D., Jessee, J. & Bloom, F.R. (1991). Plasmid transformation of *Eschericha coli* and other bacteria. *Methods in Enzymology,* 204: 63–113.

Messing, J. & Banker, A.T. (1989). The use of single-stranded DNA phage in DNA sequencing. In *Nucleic acids sequencing: A practical approach,* ed. C.J. Howe & E.S. Ward, pp. 1–36. Oxford: IRL Press.

Sambrook, J., Fritsch, E.F. & Maniatis, T. (1989). *Molecular cloning: A laboratory manual* (see especially Chapter 1). 2nd Edition, Cold Spring Harbor Laboratory Press.

Wilson, G.G. & Murray, N.E. (1991). Restriction and modification systems. *Annual Reviews of Genetics,* 25: 585–627.

Chapter 3

Banker, A.T. & Barrell, B.G. (1989). Sequencing single-stranded DNA using the chain-termination method. In *Nucleic acids sequencing: A practical approach,* ed. C.J. Howe & E.S. Ward, pp. 37–78. Oxford: IRL Press.

Huynh, T.V., Young, R.A. & Davis, R.W. (1985). Construction and screening cDNA libraries in lambda gt10 and lambda gt11. In *DNA cloning: A practical approach,* vol. 1, ed. D.M. Glover, pp. 49–78. Oxford: IRL Press.

Kaiser, K. & Murray, N.E. (1985). The use of phage lambda replacement vectors in the construction of representative genomic DNA libraries. In *DNA cloning: A practical approach*, vol. 1, ed. D.M. Glover, pp. 1–47. Oxford: IRL Press.

Messing, J. & Banker, A.T. (1989). The use of single-stranded DNA phage in DNA sequencing. In *Nucleic acids sequencing: A practical approach,* ed. C.J. Howe & E.S. Ward, pp. 1–36. Oxford: IRL Press.

Ptashne, M. (1992). *A genetic switch.* Cambridge MA: Cell Press & Blackwells.

Short, J.M., Fernandez, J.M., Sorge, J.A. & Huse, W.D. (1988). Lambda ZAP: A bacteriophage lambda expression vector with *in vivo* excision properties. *Nucleic Acids Research,* 16: 7583–7600.

Smith, G.P. & Scott, J.K. (1993). Libraries of peptides and proteins displayed on filamentous phage. *Methods in Enzymology,* 217: 228–257.

Sternberg, N.L. (1992). Cloning high molecular weight DNA fragments by the bacteriophage P1 system. *Trends in Genetics,* 8: 11–16.

Chapter 4

Davies, K.E. & Read, A.P. (1988). *Molecular basis of inherited disease.* Oxford: IRL Press.

Sambrook, J., Fritsch, E.F. & Maniatis, T. (1989). *Molecular cloning: A laboratory manual* (see especially Chapters 8 and 9). 2nd Edition, Cold Spring Harbor Laboratory Press.

Chapter 5

Davies, K.E. & Read, A.P. (1988). *Molecular basis of inherited disease.* Oxford: IRL Press.

Hediger, M.A., Coady, M.J., Ikeda, T.S. & Wright, E.M. (1987). Expression cloning and cDNA sequencing of the Na$^+$/glucose co-transporter. *Nature,* 330: 379–381.

Nierman, W.C. (1988). Vectors for cloning promoters and terminators. In *Vectors: A survey of molecular cloning vectors and their uses*, ed. R.L. Rodriguez & D.T. Denhardt, pp. 153–177. Boston: Butterworths.

Rommens, J., Iannuzzi, M.C., Kerem, B-S., Drumm, M.L., Melmer, G., Dean, M., Rozmahel, R., Cole, J.L., Kennedy, D., Hidaka, N., Zsiga, M., Buchwald, M., Riordan, J.R., Tsui, L-C. & Collins, F.S. (1989). Identification of the cystic fibrosis gene: Chromosome walking and jumping. *Science,* 245: 1059–1065.

Sambrook, J., Fritsch, E.F. & Maniatis, T. (1989). *Molecular cloning: A laboratory manual* (see especially Chapters 11 and 12). 2nd Edition, Cold Spring Harbor Laboratory Press.

Chapter 6

Goloubinoff, P., Paabo, S. & Wilson, A.C. (1993). Evolution of maize inferred from sequence diversity of an *Adh2* gene segment from archaeological remains. *Proceedings of the National Academy of Sciences of the USA*, 90: 1997–2001.

Hagelberg, E., Gray, I.C. & Jeffreys, A.J. (1991). Identification of the skeletal remains of a murder victim by DNA analysis. *Nature,* 352: 427–429.

McPherson, M.J., Quirke, P. & Taylor, G.R., eds. (1991). *PCR: A practical approach.* Oxford: IRL Press.

Saiki, R.K., Gelfand, D.H., Stoffel, S., Scharf, S.J., Higuchi, R., Horn, G.T., Mullis, K.B. & Erlich, H.A. (1988). Primer-directed enzymatic amplification of DNA with a thermostable DNA polymerase. *Science,* 239: 487–491.

Saiki, R.K., Scharf, S., Faloona, F., Mullis, K.B., Horn, G.T., Erlich, H.A. & Arnheim (1985). Enzymatic amplification of beta-globin genomic sequences and restriction site analysis for diagnosis of sickle cell anemia. *Science,* 230: 1350–1354.

Thomas, R.H., Schaffner, W., Wilson, A.C. & Paabo, S. (1989). DNA phylogeny of the extinct marsupial wolf. *Nature,* 340: 465–467.

White, T.J., Arnheim, N. & Erlich, H.A. (1989). The polymerase chain reaction. *Trends in Genetics*, 5: 185–189.

Chapter 7

Grierson, D., Fray, R.G., Hamilton, A.J., Smith, C.J.S. & Watson, C.F. (1991). Does co-suppression of sense genes in transgenic plants involve antisense RNA? *Trends in Biotechnology*, 9: 122–123.

Haseloff, J. & Gerlach, W.L. (1988). Simple RNA enzymes with new and highly specific endoribonuclease activities. *Nature,* 334: 585–591.

Rothstein, R. (1991). Targeting, disruption, replacement and allele rescue: integrative DNA transformation in yeast. *Methods in Enzymology*, 194: 281–301.

Sambrook, J., Fritsch, E.F. & Maniatis, T. (1989). *Molecular cloning: A laboratory manual* (see especially Chapter 15). 2nd Edition, Cold Spring Harbor Laboratory Press.

Smith, C.J.S., Watson, C.F., Ray, J., Bird, C.R., Morris, P.C., Schuch, W. & Grierson, D. (1988). Antisense RNA inhibition of polygalacturonase gene expression in transgenic tomatoes. *Nature,* 334: 724–726.

Symons, R.H. (1991). Ribozymes. *Critical Reviews in Plant Sciences*, 10: 189–234.

Chapter 8

Brosius, J., Erfle, M. & Storella, J. (1985). Spacing of the -10 and -35 regions in the *tac* promoter. *Journal of Biological Chemistry*, 260: 3539–3541.

Brosius, J. & Holy, A. (1984). Regulation of ribosomal RNA promoters with a synthetic *lac* operator. *Proceedings of the National Academy of Sciences of the USA*, 81: 6929–6933.

Germino, J. & Bastia, D. (1984). Rapid purification of a cloned gene product by genetic fusion and site-specific proteolysis. *Proceedings of the National Academy of Sciences of the USA*, 81: 4692–4696.

Goeddel D.V. ed. (1990). Gene expression technology. *Methods in Enzymology*, vol. 185. San Diego: Academic Press.

Krieg, P.A. & Melton, D.A. (1987). *In vitro* RNA synthesis with SP6 polymerase. *Methods in Enzymology*, 155: 397–415.

Lilius, G., Persson, M., Buflow, L. & Mosbach, K. (1991). Metal affinity precipitation of proteins carrying genetically attached polyhistidine affinity tails. *European Journal of Biochemistry*, 198: 499–504.

Nagai, K. & Thogersen, H.C. (1984). Generation of beta-globin by sequence-specific proteolysis of a hybrid protein produced in *Escherichia coli*. *Nature,* 309: 810–812.

Pelham, H.R.B. & Jackson, R.J. (1976). An efficient mRNA dependent translation system from reticulocyte lysates. *European Journal of Biochemistry*, 67: 247–256.

Chapter 9

GRAM-NEGATIVE BACTERIA

Hanahan, D., Jessee, J. & Bloom, F.R. (1991). Plasmid transformation of *Eschericha coli* and other bacteria. *Methods in Enzymology*, 204: 63–113.

Schmidhauser, T.J., Ditta, G. & Helinski, D.R. (1988). Broad host-range plasmid cloning vectors for Gram-negative bacteria. In *Vectors: A survey of molecular cloning vectors and their uses*, ed. R.L.Rodriguez & D.T. Denhardt, pp. 287–332. Boston: Butterworths.

GRAM-POSITIVE BACTERIA

Hardy, K.G. (1985). *Bacillus* cloning methods. In *DNA Cloning: A practical approach*, vol. 2, ed. D.M. Glover, pp. 1–17. Oxford: IRL Press.

Henner, D.J. (1990). Expression of heterologous genes in *Bacillus subtilis*. *Methods in Enzymology*, 185: 199–201.

Hunter, I.S. (1985). Gene cloning in *Streptomyces*. In *DNA Cloning: A practical approach*, vol. 2, ed. D.M. Glover, pp. 19–44. Oxford: IRL Press.

Le Grice, S.F.J. (1990). Regulated promoter for high-level expression of heterologous genes in *Bacillus subtilis*. *Methods in Enzymology*, 185: 201–214.

Nagarajan, V. (1990). System for secretion of heterologous proteins in *Bacillus subtilis*. *Methods in Enzymology*, 185: 214–228.

FUNGI

Punt, P.J., Oliver, R.P., Dingemanse, M.A., Pouwels, P.H. & van den Hondel, C.A.M.J.J. (1987). Transformation of *Aspergillus* based on the hygromycin B resistance marker from *Escherichia coli*. *Gene*, 56: 117–124.

Rose, M.D. & Broach, J.R. (1991). Cloning genes by complementation. *Methods in Enzymology,* 194: 195–230.

Schlessinger, D. (1990). Yeast artificial chromosomes: Tools for mapping and analysis of complex genomes. *Trends in Genetics*, 6: 248–258.

Schneider, J.C. & Guarente, L. (1991). Vectors for expression of cloned genes in yeast: Regulation, overproduction and underproduction. *Methods in Enzymology*, 194: 373–388.

Timberlake, W.E. & Marshall, M.A. (1989). Genetic engineering of filamentous fungi. *Science,* 244: 1313–1317.

Wang, J., Holden, D.W. & Leong, S.A. (1988). Gene transfer system for the phytopathogenic fungus *Ustilago maydis*. *Proceedings of the National Academy of Sciences of the USA*, 85: 865–869.

CHLAMYDOMONAS

Debuchy R., Purton, S. & Rochaix, J.-D. (1989). The argininosuccinate lyase gene of *Chlamydomonas reinhardtii*: An important tool for nuclear transformation and for correlating the genetic and molecular maps of the ARG7 locus. *EMBO Journal*, 8: 2803–2809.

Mayfield, S.P. & Kindle, K. (1990). Stable nuclear transformation of *Chlamydomonas reinhardtii* by using a *C. reinhardtii* gene as the selectable marker. *Proceedings of the National Academy of Sciences of the USA*, 87: 2087–2091.

Rochaix, J.-D., Mayfield, S., Goldschmidt-Clermont, M. & Erickson, J. (1988). Molecular biology of *Chlamydomonas*. In *Plant molecular biology: A practical approach*, ed. C.H. Shaw, pp. 253–275. Oxford: IRL Press.

VASCULAR PLANTS

Bevan, M.W. (1984). Binary *Agrobacterium* vectors for plant transformation. *Nucleic Acids Research*, 12: 8711–8721.

Croy, R.R.D., ed. (1993). *Plant Molecular Biology LABFAX*. Oxford: BIOS.

Gasser, C.S. & Fraley, R.T. (1989). Genetically engineering plants for crop improvement. *Science*, 244: 1293–1299.

Mariani, C., De Beuckleer, M., Truettner, J., Leemans, J. & Goldberg, R.B. (1990). Induction of male sterility in plants by a chimaeric ribonuclease gene. *Nature*, 347: 737–791.

Mazur, B.J. & Falco, S.C. (1989). The development of herbicide resistant crops. *Annual Reviews of Plant Physiology and Plant Molecular Biology*, 40: 441–470.

Murata, N., Ishizaki-Nishizawa, O., Higashi, S., Hayashi, H., Tasaka, Y. & Nishida, I. (1992). Genetically engineered alteration in the chilling sensitvity of plants. *Nature*, 356: 710–713.

Oeller, P.W., Min-Wong, L., Taylor, L.P., Pike, D.A. & Theologis, A. (1991). Reversible inhibition of tomato fruit senescence by antisense RNA. *Science*, 254: 437–439.

Potrykus, I. (1991). Gene transfer to plants. *Annual Reviews of Plant Physiology and Plant Molecular Biology*, 42: 205–225.

ORGANELLES

Boynton, J.E. & Gillham, N.W. (1993). Chloroplast transformation in *Chlamydomonas*. *Methods in Enzymology*, 217: 510–536.

Butow, R.A. & Fox, T.D. (1990). Organelle transformation: Shoot first, ask questions later. *Trends in Biochemical Sciences*, 15: 465–468.

Daniell, H. (1993). Foreign gene expression in chloroplasts of higher plants mediated by tungsten particle bombardment. *Methods in Enzymology*, 217: 536–556.

Folley, L.S. & Fox, T.D. (1991). Site-directed mutagenesis of a *Saccharomyces cerevisiae* mitochondrial translation initiation codon. *Genetics*, 129: 659–668.

INSECTS

Karess, R.E. (1985). P element mediated germ line transformation of *Drosophila*. In *DNA cloning: A practical approach*, vol. 2, ed. D. Glover, pp. 121–141. Oxford: IRL Press.

Kitts, P.A., Ayres, M.D., & Possee, R.D. (1990). Linearization of baculovirus DNA enhances the recovery of recombinant virus expression vectors. *Nucleic Acids Research*, 18: 5667–5672.

Lockett, T.J., Lewy, D., Holmes, P., Medveczky, K. & Saint, R. (1992). The *rough* (ro⁺) gene as a dominant P-element marker in germ line transformation of *Drosophila melanogaster. Gene,* 114: 187–193.

Luckow, V.A. & Summers, M.D. (1988). Trends in the development of baculovirus vectors. *Biotechnology,* 6: 47–55.

Pirrotta, V. (1986). Cloning *Drosophila* genes. In *Drosophila: A practical approach,* ed. D.B. Roberts, pp. 83–110. Oxford: IRL Press.

Spradling, A.C. (1986). P element–mediated transformation. In *Drosophila: A practical approach,* ed. D.B. Roberts, pp. 175–197. Oxford: IRL Press.

MAMMALS

Barnett, M.A., Buckle, V.J., Evans, E.P., Porter, A.C.G., Rout, D., Smith, A.G. & Brown, W.R.A. (1993). Telomere directed fragmentation of mammalian chromosomes. *Nucleic Acids Research,* 21: 27–36.

Bebbington, C.R. & Hentschel, C.C.G. (1987). The use of vectors based on gene amplification for the expression of cloned genes in mammalian cells. In *DNA cloning: A practical approach,* vol. 3, ed. D.M. Glover, pp. 163–188. Oxford: IRL Press.

Bueler, H., Fischer, M., Lang, Y., Bluethmann, H., Lipp, H.-P., DeArmond, S.J., Prusiner, S.B., Aguet, M. & Weissmann, C. (1992). Normal development and behaviour of mice lacking the neuronal cell-surface PrP protein. *Nature,* 356: 577–581.

Gossler, A., Joyner, A.L., Rossant, J. & Skarnes, W.C. (1989). Mouse embryonic stem cells and reporter constructs to detect developmentally regulated genes. *Science,* 244: 463–465.

Hill, D.P. & Wurst, W. (1993). Screening for novel pattern formation genes using gene trap approaches. *Methods in Enzymology,* 225: 664–681.

Kaufmann, R.J. (1990). Vectors used for expression in mammalian cells. *Methods in Enzymology,* 185: 487–511.

Mansour, S.L., Thomas, K.R. & Capecchi, M.R. (1988). Disruption of the proto-oncogene *int-2* in mouse embryo–derived stem cells: A general strategy for targeting mutations to non-selectable genes. *Nature,* 336: 348–352.

Mazzara, G.P., Destree, A. & Mahr, A. (1993). Generation and analysis of vaccinia virus recombinants. *Methods in Enzymology,* 217: 557–581.

Merlino, G.T. (1991). Transgenic animals in biomedical research. *FASEB Journal,* 5: 2996–3001.

Miller, A.D., Miller, D.G., Garcia, J.V. & Lynch, C.M. (1993). Use of retroviral vectors for gene transfer and expression. *Methods in Enzymology,* 217: 581–599.

Pursel, V.G., Pinkert, C.A., Miller, K.F., Bolt, D.J., Campbell, R.G., Palmiter, R.D., Brinster, R.L. & Hammer, R.E. (1989). Genetic engineering of livestock. *Science,* 244: 1281–1288.

Ramirez-Solis, R., Davis, A.C. & Bradley, A. (1993). Gene targeting in embryonic stem cells. *Methods in Enzymology,* 225: 855–878.

Index